Life Interrupted

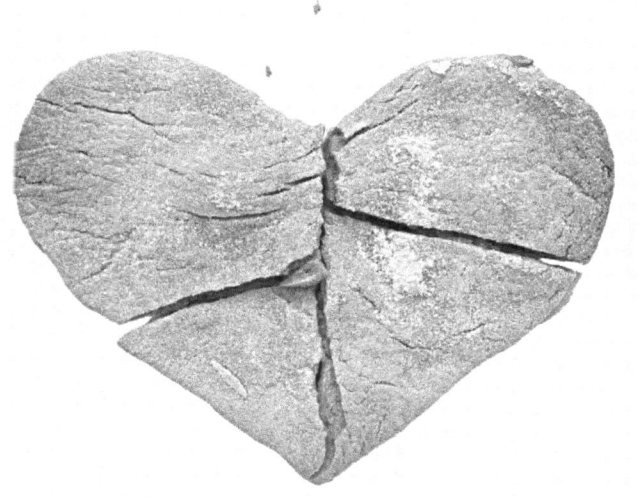

A Guide to Navigating Your
Child's Diagnosis

Zoë Rehbein

First published in Far North Queensland, 2025 by Bowerbird Publishing

© 2025 Zoë Rehbein. All rights reserved.

No part of this publication may be reproduced, stored in a retrieval system, or transmitted in any form or by any means—electronic, mechanical, photocopying, recording, or otherwise—without the prior written permission of the publisher, except in the case of brief quotations used in reviews or scholarly analysis.

This work is protected under Australian Copyright Law and international treaties.

Use of this content for the purpose of training or developing artificial intelligence (AI) systems, including large language models, machine learning, or data mining, is strictly prohibited without explicit, prior written consent from the copyright holder.

ISBN 978 1 7640739 7 4 (print)
ISBN 978 1 7640739 8 1 (ebook)

Life Interrupted
By Zoë Rehbein

Cover & Interior Design: Bowerbird Publishing
Editing: Bowerbird Publishing

Distributed by Bowerbird Publishing
Available in National Library of Australia

Disclaimer: The material in this publication is of the nature of general comment only and does not represent professional advice. It is not intended to provide specific guidance for particular circumstances. It should not be relied on as the basis of any decision to take action or not take action on any matter it covers. Readers should obtain professional advice, where appropriate, before making any such decision. To the maximum extent permitted by law, the author and publisher disclaim all responsibility and liability to any person, arising directly or indirectly from any person taking or not taking action based on the information in this publication.

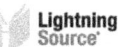

Lightning Source paper suppliers are environmentally responsible and do not use papers sourced from endangered old-growth forests, forests of exceptional conservation value, or the Amazon Basin. Lightning Source book manufacturing aims to reduce supply chain waste, greenhouse gas emissions, and conserve valuable natural resources. We share this world. We are glad to do our part in keeping it sustainable.

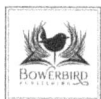

Bowerbird Publishing
Julatten, Queensland, Australia
www.crystalleonardi.com

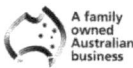 Proudly 100% Australian owned, operated & produced.

For every parent who has ever sat in a sterile room and received unthinkable news - I see you, I know you, I am you.

May you find comfort and hope within the pages of this book.

For my husband, who walks beside me with unending strength, and our three precious children - you are the heartbeat of every chapter, and the answer to every question.

"Because right now, there is someone out there with a wound in the exact shape of your words."

'Why Bother' by Sean Thomas Dougherty

CONTENTS

	About the Author	Page I
	Introduction	Page III
Chapter 1	**The Darkness of Diagnosis**	Page 1
	What is a Diagnosis?	
	A Few Stats	
	Understanding Your Child's Diagnosis	
	The Pain of Prognosis	
Chapter 2	**Liminality – The In-Between**	Page 11
Chapter 3	**Scaffolding Your New Life**	Page 13
	Building Your Team	
	Building Your New Community	
	Carer Burnout	
	Caring for Yourself	
Chapter 4	**A Whirlpool of Emotions**	Page 26
	The Grief Cycle	
	The Commonly Accepted Stages of Grief	
	Guilt - An Unwelcomed Extra	
Chapter 5	**Vulnerability Towards Courage**	Page 43
Chapter 6	**Slow Hope**	Page 49
	Finding Hope	
Chapter 7	**Navigating Relationships**	Page 54
	The Impact on Your Marriage or Partnership	
	Friendships During a Crisis	
	The Pain of Unmet Needs	
	The (Stupid) Things People Say	

Chapter 8	A Chapter For Those Who Love You Comfort In, Dump Out (The Circle of Support)	Page 72
Chapter 9	Cultivating Calm How to Process Trauma Activating the Vagus Nerve	Page 84
Chapter 10	Fear & Loss Loss	Page 96
Chapter 11	Turning to Spirituality	Page 103
Chapter 12	Grief Finding Beauty in the Broken Pieces Losing Your Child	Page 109
Chapter 13	Growth Through Trauma (Forged in Fire) How do you Process Trauma, Find Meaning From it, & Move Towards Growth?	Page 115
Chapter 14	From One Parent to Another	Page 125

Author's Note	Page 141
Appendix	Page 143
Acknowledgement	Page 147
From the Publisher	Page 153

About the Author

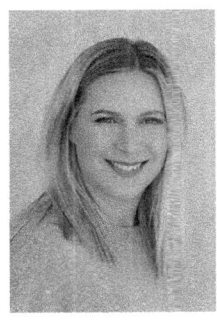
Zoë Rehbein is a writer, advocate, and mother of three whose life was forever changed when her youngest child was diagnosed with a complex medical condition. In this, her debut book, Life Interrupted: A Guide to Navigating Your Child's Diagnosis, Zoë offers a compassionate and practical roadmap for families facing the unimaginable, drawing from her lived experience and years of advocacy work with the Children's Tumour Foundation.

A passionate supporter of families navigating the medical system, Zoë has been a driving force behind community fundraising efforts, patient support initiatives, and awareness campaigns. Her tireless work has earned her recognition at both grassroots and national levels.

When she's not writing or reading, Zoë can usually be found cheering from the sidelines of a football field, or in the waiting room of a hospital—places that have become part of her rhythm as a mother and fierce advocate. She lives in Brisbane, Australia, with her husband and three children.

Zoë can be contacted on the following platforms:

www.zoerehbein.com
Instagram: @the_lifeinterrupted
Facebook: Life Interrupted
Facebook group: Life Interrupted Community

Introduction

Life interrupted. I've borrowed this phrase from a beautiful childhood cancer awareness post on social media. From the moment I read it, it stayed with me. It took my breath away. I had to pause, so I could sit with the weight of it for a moment.

Life. Interrupted.

Our daughter's life, interrupted.
Her brothers' lives, interrupted.
Dreams, interrupted.
School days, interrupted.
Peaceful nights, interrupted.
Careers, interrupted.
Happiness, interrupted.
A future, interrupted.

The diagnosis of a life-changing or life-threatening illness in a child is one of the most devastating and impactful events in a parent or caregiver's life. It can tear apart the most resilient and bring the strongest to their knees. It can make you question your faith and rob you of hope for the future.

A diagnosis has the potential to upend your life in a way you could never have foreseen, touching every corner of your soul, and every area of your life. I often refer to the experience of having a critically or chronically unwell child, as operating from deep within the trenches, where everything is so very difficult and suddenly the world around us (and above us) feels foreign. We bunker down and focus on survival.

The trauma of having a sick child leaves an imprint on us all, and without appropriate support and care that trauma becomes embedded, manifesting in sickness, grief and relentless stress.

10 years ago, our lives were torn apart when our baby girl was diagnosed with a rare and complex genetic disorder, Neurofibromatosis type 1 (NF1). She was just 9 weeks old. I sat in shock as the specialist outlined what we might expect for her future, detailing a world in which tumours, both benign and malignant, would grow within her little body, anywhere there are nerves, including the brain and spine. As the weight of his words settled upon me, the lights dimmed, and I sat alone in my loss. The very essence of me simply faded away. I had been given 9 perfect weeks with my beautiful girl before the lights went out.

The slow burn of grief imprinted itself on my soul, changing who I was and what I believed in. It was in the shadow of my smile, in the curve of my mouth, in the lines around my eyes, and in the depths of my heart. I longed for someone to save her, without realising it was me who needed to be saved. She was as perfect as she had always been.

The pain I felt was unending, and the unexpected weight of guilt was unbearable. I forgot how to do the simplest of things, like scrambling eggs. Everyday tasks, like opening the curtains in the morning, felt pointless. In one fell swoop the laughter had died on my lips, and my words had simply stopped. I couldn't speak. I couldn't write

I alternated between feeling lost and bereft, and fighting an overwhelming sense of panic. I would research all day and night, trying to find the loophole that would allow my daughter to escape the future we'd been told awaited her. And when there wasn't one to be found, all I could do was cry. The darkness was like a weighty cloak upon my shoulders, grounding me, turning me in upon myself.

When our beautiful girl turned two, our fears were realised, and she was diagnosed with brain and spinal tumours and, shortly after, with a tumour in her arm. Over the past seven years, she has undergone numerous rounds of chemotherapy and targeted cancer treatments. As a family, we've navigated these challenging times together, learning to balance strength and courage with fear, while holding tight to the joy and love that we share. And there really has been so much love and happiness. So much growth.

Partway through writing this book our girl began treatment again, this time with a new and promising targeted drug, and I was reminded all over again of the grief of diagnosis. I felt again the lingering sense of panic and would lie awake in bed with a familiar tightness in my chest. I was reminded that you never get over a diagnosis. You don't get used to hearing bad news or fear the unknown any less.

But you do develop a resilience along the way that allows you to carry the weight of the experience a little better. You learn that it's a lonely journey and while there is no one on this planet who truly knows what you're going through, you begin to understand that parents walking the same, or similar, path as you are your lifeline. You collect a few little tools along the way that lessen the horror and dull the panic. You remember to breathe. You remember to be kind to yourself. You find the glimmers of joy that exist within the painful moments, and you hold them tight.

This is the book I wished for when I was going through my most painful moments at the beginning of our medical journey. A book of acknowledgement, of support, of hope and love. Some gentle suggestions, some practical guides, and most of all, understanding. I didn't have the energy or the inclination to trawl through dozens of books to find a ray of hope, and toxic positivity broke me. I couldn't focus on anything heavy and difficult. I just needed a single book, like a warm embrace, to gently carry me through. A book that I could open at any page and take what I needed in the moment.

This is that book. What this isn't is my daughter's story. That's hers to tell if or when she chooses, to whomever she chooses. This is my experience in relation to her diagnosis, and my learnings from the past decade.

I hope 'Life Interrupted' carries you through your moments of heartbreak and comforts you when it all feels too much. I hope it feels like safe hands reaching down to you, pulling you up and out of the trenches when you just can't manage it alone.

I also hope it sees you all the way through to the other side—not necessarily of the illness or the diagnosis, but of your growth and evolution—towards resilience and joy in the face of heartache. Because no matter where you are today, your feelings will change, they will evolve, and you will get through this. And as Bono says, joy is the ultimate act of defiance.

One day at a time. One moment at a time. Gently, gently.

Disclaimer: This book is not intended as a guide to navigating the loss of a child. While it may acknowledge and reflect on that experience, its primary focus is on the broader journey of parenting a critically or chronically ill child. If you are grieving the loss of your child, please know you are not alone. There are dedicated resources and professionals who can support you through this unimaginable time. Please reach out to your GP, psychologist, social worker, or nurse for guidance to the support services best suited to your needs.

CHAPTER 1
The Darkness of Diagnosis

Every moment of every day, someone, somewhere, is receiving a diagnosis for their child of a life-changing, life-altering, or life-threatening nature. Because you're reading this book, I'm assuming that one of those moments was yours, and one of those diagnoses was your child's. And I'm so sorry that's happened to your child, to you, and to your family. You may have seen the diagnosis coming, or it may have come as a complete shock. Either way, how you're feeling in this moment is completely unique. No one has stood in your shoes, with your child, in this exact moment, hearing these words.

In an ideal world, I hope the diagnosis was delivered to you carefully, with full recognition of the impact and momentousness of the news. I hope the doctor giving the diagnosis sat gently with your shock and your grief and held space for your pain.

Realistically, we're often delivered the news in a clinical setting, with shock underpinning every word. It can be difficult to understand what's being said, what it means, and what the future holds. Your heart and your brain are in disconnect, and you don't have the right words, or the right questions, in the moment.

Often, once the shock wears off and the reality sets in, we find ourselves with a thousand conflicting thoughts and emotions. Sharing with family and friends can make it feel even more real, and their questions may feel overwhelming, when you haven't yet had a chance to consider those questions yourself. You may not have answers for everyone, and that's okay. The answers will come.

It's completely normal to feel all the emotions right now, and the most important thing is that you give yourself the grace and the space to feel them all. You may feel confused or angry, desperate and panicked. You may find yourself sitting in blankness or crying uncontrollably. You may want to call everyone you know just to say the words out loud. Or perhaps the idea of speaking those words out loud, even softly, is inconceivable.

A shock diagnosis, or a diagnosis in any form, hits us all differently.

If you're someone who needs space to process, take that space. In this first instance, place a gentle boundary around your heart and your mind, and step away from the noise. This might look like moving into another room, to think or to cry, or taking a long shower or having a warm bath.

If you're a people person, surround yourself with those who will come to you in support, in whatever way you need. I've been in hospital rooms filled with family and friends, bringing noise and hope and comfort. And I've sat in the quiet grief of a darkened room, where the effort to speak is too much.

What is a Diagnosis?

A diagnosis is the process of identifying an illness, condition, disease or injury based on medical symptoms, medical history and tests such as scans and blood tests. Once a name can be given to the health issue it becomes easier to identify an approach to treatment and management. Sometimes the process of diagnosis can be long and excruciating, and at other times it comes quickly and unexpectedly.

As a parent, you will receive innumerable diagnoses for your children throughout their childhood, and most will be unpleasant but easily managed. Some of the most common childhood diagnoses include asthma, Ear, Nose and Throat (ENT) issues, gastrointestinal issues, developmental and learning disorders (such as autism spectrum disorder (ASD), and Attention-Deficit Hyperactivity Disorder (ADHD), amongst others.

Less commonly, children are diagnosed with serious conditions or diseases that have the potential to uproot life as you know it. While less common, these conditions have significant impacts and may require long term management or invasive treatments.

The diagnosis of a serious condition in your child is one of the most life-altering experiences you will ever face, and I extend my most heartfelt condolences that this is happening to you and to the child you love. Truly, I am so sorry.

Some of the most common serious childhood diagnoses include
- Cancer – most commonly leukaemia, brain and central nervous system tumours, and lymphoma.

- Congenital heart defects
- Cystic fibrosis (CF)
- Type 1 diabetes
- Epilepsy
- Sickle cell disease
- Muscular dystrophy (MD)
- Cerebral palsy (CP)
- Spinal muscular atrophy (SMA)
- Severe autism spectrum disorder (ASD)
- Inflammatory bowel disease (IBD)
- Severe mental health disorders
- Genetic disorders with developmental impacts
- Rett syndrome, and
- Neurodegenerative disorders

Sadly, this is by no means an exhaustive list, and many additional serious childhood conditions exist. These conditions often require multidisciplinary care, symptom management and support services, to help your child lead their best life while supporting the families impacted. They can also enormously impact families, creating isolation, lost income, and a greatly altered future.

A Few Stats

Approximately 1 in 12 babies worldwide are born with a rare disease. There are over 7,000 rare diseases, a few of which are on the list above, and around 75% of these affect children.[1]

---

[1] Murdoch Children's Research Institute, Rare Disease Flagship.

The prevalence of rare diseases in children is a significant global concern, with implications on healthcare systems, families and communities. While rare diseases are individually uncommon, collectively they affect millions of children worldwide, highlighting the need for improved awareness, timely diagnosis and effective treatments. Importantly, they affect millions of families worldwide, with parents and siblings facing into a difficult and unknown future, often feeling unprepared and isolated.

While medical professionals, medical journals, and information sources bandy around statistics, when it's your child, your diagnosis, and your life, a statistic is meaningless. Regardless of whether there is a 1 in 3,000 chance or 1 in a million chance of your child's diagnosis, when your child is the ONE, these statistics mean very little.

I grew up in a small town of roughly 4,000 people. When my little one was first diagnosed, I used to imagine them all standing together, facing me. Within that enormous group of people, statistically speaking, only one of them would have been diagnosed with NF. I tortured myself with that visual. Out of thousands of people, my baby girl was the one. I would imagine her standing apart from the collective, facing into her future alone, and it broke my heart.

At times I would attempt to work out how many babies were born in Australia on the day my daughter was born, then how many that month, then how many that year. For those playing along at home, those numbers were something like 821, 24,972, and 299,700. That equates to roughly 100 babies that year being born with NF, or nine per month, across Australia. Then I narrowed my search to the hospital she was born in. I discovered that in the year 2014, 9,838 babies were born in that hospital, and of those, just three in that entire year would have been born with NF. She was one of just three.

Sometimes I would wonder how the other mothers were coping. If they were as broken as I was.

Was all this searching helpful? No. Was it comforting? Not remotely. I'm not entirely sure what I was looking for, but it was a necessary part of my processing, and a painful part of my grief journey.

Understanding Your Child's Diagnosis

Almost immediately following a diagnosis, you'll need to understand what you and your child are facing. When staring into an uncertain future, the lure of Google can be strong (and it has its place). However, most doctors will caution against turning to the internet for medical information. Depending on the diagnosis your child has received, there may not be information available online that is specific to your child, and you may read information that needlessly creates more fear and greater confusion.

Putting together a list of questions to ask your medical practitioner can be a helpful first step in understanding your child's individual and unique situation. These questions should broadly cover the themes of understanding the diagnosis, understanding treatment options, and understanding what comes next, today and into the future. It can be useful to bring someone with you to act as an extra pair of ears, to take notes, and refer to them later.

At the back of this book, I've included a list of questions to bring along to your medical appointment (Appendix). Please feel free to personalise this list and add or remove questions as appropriate.

The Pain of Prognosis

When we think of prognosis, we often think of the end stages of someone's life. However, a prognosis is simply a doctor's prediction regarding the likely course, duration, and outcome of your child's condition or illness. It considers the severity of the condition, the expected progression, and any chance of recovery or remission, while considering possible complications. If your child's condition is very serious it may include an estimate of life expectancy.

Understanding your child's prognosis can be helpful for families while also being extremely painful. A prognosis allows you to set realistic expectations on the expected course of the illness and identifies possible challenges and outcomes—which can be helpful in preparing for what lies ahead, both practically and emotionally.

It's important to remember that a prognosis is not exact and is based on many factors, including overall health and available treatment options. However, it provides a general guide to help parents and families prepare, plan and make decisions.

It's also useful to remember that sometimes a medical specialist may be reluctant or unable to provide a prognosis until they have more information. Similarly, if you would rather not know your child's prognosis, it's vital that you communicate that to your medical team.

When I asked our nurse why our treating specialist hadn't given us a prognosis, her response really moved me. She said, "Because sometimes a prognosis can steal hope, and hope is so very powerful. Hope can change everything."

A note for the broken hearted,

Her diagnosis was the greatest thief.

It crept in when she was a wisp of a child and stole something from me that I will never get back. An innocence that I cannot reclaim.

It stole something that I hadn't even realised I thought was mine – the certainty that our precious baby girl would have a wonderful life.

The certainty that she would crawl, walk, run, talk, love us, and be loved by us. The certainty that she was ours to keep.

With her diagnosis I lost the magic of those early days with my sweet baby

I lost joy, I lost hope, I lost heart. Without an outlet for my anger, I directed it straight at the 'chances' of this happening to her, and I lost faith in the comfort of statistics.

The only somewhat comforting thing is that she was too little to remember any of the painful early months after her diagnosis. She has no memory of the tears that fell on her sweet little head as I fed her, or of the many words fiercely whispered to her in the dark of the night, words of grief and fear and apology. Of mummy whispering 'I'm so sorry' over and over again, until it resembled the soothing 'shush shush' sounds I should've been making.

She won't remember the doctor's first shocking explanations, the questions, or the tears. She won't remember that Mummy couldn't get up, couldn't breathe, couldn't leave the hospital car park. She won't remember how I broke into a thousand tiny pieces, wanting to tear the skin that no longer fit from my broken body.

And for all that, if nothing else, I am grateful.

You can do this,

Love, Me x

CHAPTER 2
Liminality - The In-Between

In liminality, time becomes suspended between the before and after. You're not the parent you were before diagnosis, and yet you're not the person you'll become. You are in limbo, navigating a lonely and painful experience without certainty of the outcome. This is not the life you knew, or the one you expected.

Liminality is the gap between the words, the blank line between the paragraphs. It's the in-between, where you've left one chapter and are waiting for the next to begin. The chapter where you emerge stronger.

In the before, life held a predictable and ordinary rhythm. You had assurance of what lay ahead. There were school drop-offs, dinners to be made, school sports, and stories at bedtime. There were nappies to be changed, bottles of formula to be given, nights spent rocking a baby to sleep. In the before, you knew what needed to be done.

In the after, nothing is recognisable. All familiarity has been stripped away. Now you're a caregiver, medical researcher, nurse, advocate. You speak a new language—one of bloods and treatment protocols. There is no certainty and some days you're sleepwalking through the experience.

Who are you now, in this in-between space? What have you become?

The liminal space is isolating. Friends post about milestones, normal events, holidays, while you blink slowly to the sound of a beeping monitor. Time has no meaning here, in the in-between. A day is either a 'good' day or a 'bad' day now, depending on test results or doctors' consultations. All of it outside of your control. You see others in the same liminal space, faces carefully blank in the waiting rooms and hospital corridors. There's a quiet solidarity between you. You're in the in-between together.

Your nerves are taut with tension. You hover between the states of fear and hope, dread and bravery. There is no certainty. Some days you ride high on quiet hope and optimism, and on others, you're washed away in a wave of despair.

You wonder how this will end. Or if it ever will. And so, you exist in the in-between, parenting with a fierce, protective love. You speak your new language and learn to lean into your new life. Quietly evolving and growing, you redefine your life—until one day, you realise you've emerged from the in-between and are in the next chapter—one of healing and growth. And your strength, intertwined with tenderness and exhaustion, is nothing short of beautiful.

CHAPTER 3
Scaffolding Your New Life

Building Your Team

At this stage of the journey, you'll have discussed your child's diagnosis with your clinician and should have a clearer idea of whether they have a treatment plan—and if so, what it entails. You'll know which specialists make up your medical team and how involved they are likely to be in managing your child's condition. While you'll have a managing medical specialist, it's not uncommon to have several different practitioners from various medical fields checking in less frequently. For example, your child may need yearly eye tests, respiratory tests, or visits to specialised clinics such as a pain or sleep clinics.

Your medical team may also include allied health professionals. Allied health professionals work alongside doctors, nurses and families to provide holistic care for your child. They provide support in hospital, in the community, and at home—focusing on your child's health, wellbeing, and rehabilitation (if required). Some examples of allied health professionals include:

Physiotherapists

When a Physiotherapist works with your child, their goal is to improve mobility, strength, and coordination that may have been affected by your child's condition. A physiotherapist also supports children with physical disabilities or developmental delays by helping them develop gross motor skills. They play a major role in rehabilitation after surgery and work closely with you and your child to regain and maintain movement and function.

Occupational Therapists (OT's)

An Occupational Therapist (OT) will work with families to help their child develop or regain skills that are needed for everyday life, such as eating, playing or dressing themselves. It may be hard to comprehend that your child needs this kind of support; however, during treatment, after surgery or in times of disease progression, your child may find everyday tasks difficult.

Your child plays many important roles in life—as a learner, family member, student, friend, and more. When they take on the new role of 'patient', these existing roles can be disrupted. An OT helps children navigate this challenge by tailoring therapy to their individual needs, whether they're living with Autism, cancer, or another condition. The goal is to support the child in continuing to participate in all aspects of life, while also managing the responsibilities that come with their condition—like taking medication or undergoing medical procedures. Therapy may focus on building fine motor skills, developing strategies for emotional regulation, or modifying tasks and environments to promote independence in daily activities. This might include learning how to manage their own schedule or using special cutlery to make mealtimes easier.

In a hospital setting, an OT plays a key role in helping your child understand their condition and what to expect during their stay—all in an age-appropriate and supportive way. They help prepare children for medical procedures and provide emotional support throughout the journey. For younger children, this might involve creating a personalised storybook using simple language and photos of the hospital environment and medical team, to explain what will happen in a way that feels safe and familiar.

Throughout treatment, your OT will monitor your child's development and support them in staying connected to their everyday roles—whether that's keeping in touch with friends, staying engaged with school, or simply playing. They can also provide support for siblings, helping them understand what's going on and addressing any concerns or fears they may have.

If you think your child would benefit from OT support during their hospital stay, speak to your medical team about connecting with a hospital-based OT. OTs are also available in the community to provide ongoing support at home or in a clinic. Your care team may be able to recommend someone, or you might ask other parents or a support group for a trusted referral

Building Your New Community

There is nothing lonelier, in the liminal realm, than the early days of diagnosis. When you no longer know who you are, who you need to be, or how you'll navigate this terrifying new world. Seeking out others who can genuinely understand and empathise with you is critical. Other parents with lived experience can offer both practical and emotional support. They might be the parents you bump into in the waiting room, or while making a coffee in the family room, or the ones you find in online groups. However it happens, seeking those connections is so crucial to your emotional health moving forward.

The first step towards connection, is to search online for an organisation that represents your child's condition or illness. These organisations often have online support, and depending on the size of the organisation may also have in-person support available. They may run social media groups where you can connect with others, or host virtual meet-ups, counselling groups, or peer support sessions. Many organisations offer phone calls with a counsellor or support worker who can gently hold your hand through the especially difficult moments, and offer the comfort and tools needed to carry you through. They may also be able to connect you with other parents and families walking a similar medical path.

In 2016, one of the world's leading journals in paediatrics, Developmental Medicine and Child Neurology, published a study that found that parent-to-parent support significantly decreased symptoms of anxiety and depression among parents of children with complex medical conditions. The study reported that parents who participated in peer support had higher levels of emotional resilience and reported greater self-efficacy, meaning they felt more confident and capable of handling the challenges associated with their child's diagnosis.

A growing body of research supports this conclusion, showing that peer support has a significant effect on a parent's ability to cope with the stress of caring for a seriously or critically ill child. It improves mental health, reduces stress, decreases anxiety and depression, lessens feelings of isolation, enhances resilience, and empowers parents to advocate for their child.

While it might feel like all you want to do is stick your head in the sand, connecting with others when your child is diagnosed can be the difference between coping and not coping. Parents in the same boat, particularly those further into their child's health journey, can often offer coping strategies and support on those days when you're struggling. They can offer a unique form of emotional support that others will not be able to provide. This is because they understand the specific fears, worries and hopes that come with your child's diagnosis, without you needing to offer extensive explanations. As such, they often show a level of empathy and compassion that, try as they might, family and friends can't always offer. These connections help reduce stress, decrease feelings of anxiety, and improve mental wellbeing by offering a safe space to share fears and concerns.

Medical parents are also a wealth of information. They can offer practical tips to navigating the healthcare system, treatment options and side effects, clinical trials and how to access resources. No-one knows their child's condition better than a medical parent.

They'll often be your go-to for information regarding education adjustments, financial hardship supports, foundations, therapies and more.

Being a part of a community—albeit it one you never asked to join—can be empowering at a time when you feel lost. It can provide structure for how to share information online, how to communicate with family and friends, how to explain the condition, and how to advocate for your child. You might find yourself drawn to fundraising or awareness opportunities, which can offer purpose and meaning. Taking action, even in small ways, can help to alleviate feelings of helplessness and give you a sense of direction.

Tip: Search online for an organisation or charity that represents your child's condition. If you're uncertain, ask your medical professional or a nurse, or delegate the task to a friend who's looking for ways to help.

Carer Burnout

Carer burnout is a state of emotional, physical, and mental exhaustion that arises from caring for a child with medical complexities. Recent research highlights the considerable impact of carer fatigue—or burnout—on parents who care for children with serious illnesses. This often differs significantly from 'normal' parental stress (which is difficult in its own right), both in its intensity and complexity.

Where parental burnout arises from the routine stresses of work life balance, family demands, and loss of personal time—combined with emotions such as frustration, fatigue and guilt—carer burnout takes this to the next level. The parent of a medically complex or unwell child continues to carry their responsibilities as a parent, partner, employee, friend, daughter or son, while also managing the intense physical, logistical, and emotional demands of caring for their child.

Carers of unwell children often face heightened stress due to constant health concerns, frequent hospital visits, and managing complex medical routines. Their daily tasks can be relentlessly demanding, involving the administration of medications, medical treatments, or procedures—alongside the pressures of running a household and maintaining family schedules. This can also include disrupted sleep: for instance, giving overnight medications or soothing their child—regardless of the child's age. The strain intensifies when other young children in the home also require care during the night. Over time, this creates deep emotional fatigue, with feelings of grief, helplessness, and trauma layered over an ever-present sense of existential worry—feelings not typically associated with standard parental burnout.

Social isolation can further compound carer fatigue. While parents may crave normalcy and connection through social outings, their child's condition—such as being immunocompromised or medically fragile—can make participation impossible. Families may be forced into isolation to protect their child's health. This leads to a deep sense of disconnection, with few opportunities to recharge or feel understood by those outside the medical parenting world.

Medical parents must be mindful of the long-term impact of sustained stress and anxiety. Chronic exhaustion and fear for their child's future are linked to poor psychological outcomes and can increase the risk of developing long-term mental health conditions.

While mental health challenges such as depression and anxiety are not unique to medical parents, the context of their stress often is. For parents of unwell children, the primary stressor—their child's health—cannot be removed. This makes it much harder to find resolution, closure, or peace of mind. The weight of this becomes even heavier in cases involving intensive care routines, such as diabetes, cerebral palsy, or cancer, or when navigating a lifelong diagnosis.

A systematic review published in the Journal of Paediatric Psychology was the first of its kind to examine the stress experienced by parents caring for children with a wide range of conditions— including asthma, cancer, cystic fibrosis, diabetes, epilepsy, juvenile rheumatoid arthritis and, sickle cell disease. The review identified key stressors that exacerbate carer stress, including:

- The responsibility of managing a chronically ill child's medical care.
- Integrating the sick child's needs into the family routine.
- Coordinating schooling for their sick child.
- Watching their child in pain.
- Explaining their child's health problems to others.[2]

---

[2] https://evidencebasedliving.human.cornell.edu/blog/new-evidence-on-the-stress-of-parenting-sick-children

Other major contributors to burnout include financial strain, difficulty balancing work and family life, and unpredictable or disrupted daily routines. In many families, one parent takes on the primary role of caregiver, while the other becomes the financial provider. This divide can leave both parents feeling isolated, unsupported, and overwhelmed in different ways.

Connecting with others facing similar challenges can ease anxiety and reduce the sense of isolation. Sharing fears and experiences within a safe, understanding community can help you connect with appropriate resources and support—and restore a sense of hope and resilience for the road ahead.

Caring for Yourself

One of the most frustrating things I am consistently asked by others is what I'm doing to care for myself. I'll be honest, there are times when the concept is almost laughable.

This question in itself is a tricky one. I'm sure it comes from a good place, but it may not always come across that way. Asking this question of the parent of an unwell child can foster a sense of shame—shame that we're somehow failing to adequately look after ourselves, shame that the inadequacy has been noted, and shame that we're clearly not balancing the demands of this life as well as others might.

It also subtly implies that the asker has no idea what you're going through, which can feel isolating and diminishing.

I think we're all aware of the old, 'put your own mask on first' analogy; however, there are times when the focus is more on keeping your head above water—on simply continuing to exist in a foreign and difficult world, to the best of your ability. There will be days when you won't have the energy to apply your own mask, and the very idea of undertaking self-care on top of everything else is ludicrous. I've often joked that my mantra since this began has been: 'Surviving is thriving.'

During our medical journey, there have been times when a shower every second day was considered self-care. There are times I have cried every day, left my emails to accumulate to horrifying levels, and stopped answering the phone. I've read important school correspondence four months after the fact and avoided the stack of letters on the kitchen bench—all of which made my situation feel even more overwhelming. I've since learned that this avoidance is a key indicator of emotional and mental burnout and is incredibly common when going through persistent trauma.

And then there have been times where I've had more space for self-care—where I've seen a counsellor, begun to exercise again, and have fallen asleep while listening to a sleep meditation. Days when I did far more than simply survive.

I've gone through periods of sleeping in 20-minute bursts, getting up at night to change feeding pumps, administer medications, and hold my beautiful girl who needed me. And I've gone through times when sleep hasn't been as much of an issue.

The point is that, at any given time during this journey, you will be doing the best you can with what you have. Your ability to prioritise or find space for self-care is completely dependent upon the intensity of the moment you are in. And as a parent of a chronically or critically unwell child, I'm going to hazard a guess that your child is currently your priority.

Having said all that—when you can, if you can—try to carve out little pieces of time for the things that matter to you. Micro-moments of self-care. It might be a bath, or going for a run, or having your nails done. It might be time to cry in the shower uninterrupted, or time to attend your other children's sporting matches and cheer from the sidelines. It might be bigger still – a weekend away, or time to go to the gym several times a week. But whatever you do, don't let anyone add self-care to the bucket of things you worry about. That bucket is already full.

A story for the one who's afraid,

When my first child was just little, we took a family holiday to Byron Bay. I stood in the shallows of the water holding him, letting the waves swirl around my knees. So happy. Perfectly content.

Suddenly, without warning, a rogue wave came through that was stronger than the others, and it knocked me over. I fell under the water, and felt my sweet boy pulled under with me. I held onto him, fiercely, but the wave was stronger than I was, and shockingly, without warning, he slipped from my fingers. Lost to me for a fraction of a second.

Completely lost. Time stood still.

And then, my fingers found him again, desperate, panicked, grabbing at his tiny limbs, grasping for him. We both rose to the surface, the same way we had fallen, with him safely tucked into my arms.

I was terrified, living and reliving the moment he left my hands and was lost to me. But to the outside world, nothing had happened at all.

When I think of childhood illness, of brain tumours that are quietly simmering but momentarily stable, this is what I come back to. It's holding onto my girl as though my life depends on it, watching and waiting for the wave that could sweep her away.

It's torn fingernails and aching jaws and never letting my guard down. It's falling and fighting, then rising to the surface with no one any the wiser as to what happened beneath the water. It's the enormous sense of loss as my fingers clutch thin air for a moment or two. It's hoping that my love is strong enough to fight against a force that's greater than I am. It's the fear of what's coming.

It's watching the tide ebb out to sea, the sands becoming exposed and naked, not knowing if the next wave will be the one that will sweep me off my feet. And my hands will come up empty.

I see you.
Me x

CHAPTER 4
A Whirlpool of Emotions

The Grief Cycle

The diagnosis of your child can be a deeply disruptive and traumatic experience. You may experience a maelstrom of feelings, often in unpredictable and rapid succession, ranging from calm and accepting, to almost violently disbelieving or angry. Sometimes these emotions can catch us by surprise, however, gaining an understanding of the complexity of your emotional response can help you to move through the emotions in a more compassionate way.

The Grief Cycle, or the five stages of grief, was first coined by psychiatrist Elisabeth Kübler-Ross in her 1969 book 'On Death and Dying.' Originally, the stages referred to the emotional journey of the terminally ill, however, over time it has been applied more broadly to a range of situations where grief is the main character.

The Grief Cycle identifies five key emotions that come with a grief journey – denial, anger, bargaining, depression, and acceptance. While many people feel this encapsulates the experience well, others may feel it simplifies the grief process. It is, however, a useful framework to talk about and better understand our emotions.

It's also important to remember that there is no rule book accompanying these stages. You may experience these emotions in a completely non-linear fashion, jumping wildly between depression and anger, or oscillating between denial and acceptance. Similarly, bargaining might be something you do over and over, or it may not be a big focus for you.

When it comes to the grief associated with a childhood diagnosis, the emotions most expressed to me have been fear, panic, and guilt. While these are powerful emotions, they are each encapsulated within the original five stages of grief, even though they very often feel they should have their own category… in capital letters and flashing lights.

It can be difficult to navigate the stages of grief when those close to you would like you to move on from the emotional stage you're currently experiencing. Encouraging you to move towards acceptance is well-meaning but misguided, and ultimately leads to a sense of shame that you're not coping with the situation as well as you might.

Tip: Pre-empt well-meaning encouragement to move through your emotions by coming up with a comeback line. A comeback line is a pre-prepared one-line response to commonly posed thoughts or questions. For example, your friend tells you it would be easier for you if you could find some acceptance of the situation. Your response might be as simple as, "I'm just not there yet," or "Thank you for thinking of me," or "I'm taking this one day at a time." What you're doing is closing the conversation, which is often what you need most in that moment.

As we walk this path together, you'll notice a recurrent theme – grief is a deeply personal journey, and your experience will be like no other. There is no right or wrong way to experience this diagnosis, or what comes next. Even people closest to you and your child - your partner, your mum or your best friend - are unlikely to experience this in the same way you are. As painful as it is, this journey is yours, and yours alone. They have their own path to walk.

The Commonly Accepted Stages of Grief

1. Denial

It's not uncommon to enter a state of denial when your child is first diagnosed, and again at various intervals throughout your journey. If your child's journey involves multiple stages of treatment, or periods of change, denial can continue to pop up along the way.

Though denial often carries negative connotations, it serves a vital and necessary purpose—it shields your heart and mind from the initial shock of diagnosis, gently easing you into an unfamiliar and frightening new world.

Denial may show up as a refusal to accept the diagnosis, and you may choose to seek out second or third opinions. If you have the time and capacity to do this, it's not a bad idea. Others may find acceptance of the news difficult and not share it with the people who love and support them.

Inevitably, denial is a short-term emotion, and often the necessity of dealing with the situation will propel you forward in your emotional journey. Staying in denial too long could delay important decision-making, or the commencement of treatments, which might be necessary for your child.

2. Anger

When a diagnosis is unexpected or life altering, anger is a very common response.

Anger often masks a sub-set of deeper and more uncomfortable emotions that we may struggle to articulate, or that lead us deeper into despair. It's far easier to say "I'm angry" than it is to delve into fear, uncertainty or injustice. The loss of control and sense of powerlessness is deepened in the context of a parent's biological and primal need to keep their child safe. The realisation that your child's well-being may be outside of your control can be devastating.

The uncertainty of the moment you are in, and the implications for the future, can also trigger anger. Anger is a familiar way to cope with the overwhelming thoughts you may be facing – fearing suffering, difficulty or even death – and can also represent a deep sense of injustice or unfairness at the situation.

Some people may become stuck on the difficult question "why them?", letting that thought fester and grow until they feel nothing but anger for those who aren't in their situation. You may feel angry that no-one else understands what you're facing or feeling. Or angry that a God or universal being could inflict such pain upon a child.

To combat these feelings, some people find it helpful to ask the question "Why not me?", implying a sense of randomness, and that it could just as easily happen to them as to someone else. I think this question requires a level of acceptance that often comes further down the track. It may also help to lean more heavily towards your religion or belief system for support, rather than rail against it.

Anger can also be an expression of grief and loss. When the diagnosis jeopardises the life that you thought your child would have, your hopes and dreams for their future, or the future you had envisioned for your family, it's natural to feel an element of anger.

Tip: Try not to make anger the enemy. Recognise it for what it is — a masking emotion for deeper, more difficult emotions. Say them out loud and acknowledge that they exist. You're going to need to get comfortable with a whole raft of different emotions

3. Bargaining

Bargaining is a common response to a child's diagnosis, particularly in the early stages.

Bargaining often involves making internal deals or pleas in a desperate attempt to regain control over an uncontrollable situation. It stems from a powerful need to protect your child or to somehow make the diagnosis disappear.

Bargaining might look like:
- Internal Promises: Parents may make promises to a higher power, themselves, or their child, such as, "If my child gets better, I will do everything differently," or, "I will be a better person if this treatment works."

- If/Then Thinking: Bargaining is often characterized by thoughts like, "If only I had caught this earlier, then maybe this wouldn't have happened," or "If we try one more treatment, then everything will turn out okay."
- Guilt and Regret: Some parents bargain with their own sense of guilt, thinking about what they could have done differently to prevent the diagnosis. This may involve bargaining with "what-ifs" or regretting past decisions, even if they had no control over the outcome. It often sparks thoughts of wanting a do-over, to correct perceived mistakes. What this is really doing is laying blame at your own feet, which can feel easier than having no-one to blame at all.

Bargaining is a painful stage in the Grief Cycle but is often the first step in moving towards acceptance. Bargaining offers a temporary reprieve from the helplessness you may be feeling and allows you to momentarily avoid the weight of your emotions. Coming to terms with the thought that a child's illness is outside of your control will help you facilitate moving through this painful stage.

Tip: Connecting with support networks, such as networks specifically relating to your child's diagnosis can really help contextualise your pain and support you in moving forward. In addition, turning towards your faith, for those who are religious or spiritual, can often provide great comfort.

4. Depression

Depression often emerges a little later, as the gravity of the situation becomes apparent, and you begin to accept that this is in fact happening. Unlike Clinical Depression, which is a long-term mental health condition, depression in the context of grief is often situational. It's an understanding and a realisation of the situation you are in.

Depression is often a sadder, more resigned reaction to the emotions that had previously been present under the guise of anger. Without the mask of anger, depression allows you to process your emotions more deeply and more genuinely. It's a realisation of loss, a sense of hopelessness, and a feeling of being overwhelmed by just how much life has changed. It may feel like a deep-seated sadness, and tears may be forever close to the surface. Or it may feel like a sense of emptiness, or a well of tiredness that you can't overcome. Depression comes in many guises, which also means it can be hard for the people around you to recognise the signs.

The depression stage is difficult for parents and caregivers to move through. It can often lead to withdrawal from friends and from activities you'd previously engaged in, which can lead to isolation and a worsening sense of loss. If you're struggling through this stage, it's critical that you reach out to friends, family or trained professionals to help you navigate through this emotion. Coming to terms with your grief and sense of loss can feel like a dark period, but acknowledging your feelings is an important step towards healing, allowing you to better cope with what's happening.

5. Acceptance

More than any other stage, parents and caregivers often struggle with this stage the most. And yet it's the emotional plateau that those who love us the most are desperate for us to stand upon. Away from rage and denial and depression. Away from pleading and bargaining with the universe. Away from loss, and pain and the ugliness of the situation. And towards the hint of a smile, and a glimmer of light.

However, it can often feel unreasonable to be expected to find acceptance in the face of an unexpected diagnosis. I felt like I was being asked to accept the inconceivable, to accept the unfairness and the grief and the pain. There were days I could barely breathe; such was the weight pressing upon my chest. I wanted to tear at my body, perhaps to redirect the emotional pain to a physical one that I could understand, or maybe to visually demonstrate the enormous pain within my heart.

Being asked to accept my daughter's diagnosis before I was ready sparked rage within me. Every cell in my body railed against it, fighting against a state of defeat. I felt that moving into this stage would mean accepting that our daughter's life was going to be painful, and traumatic, and that I could lose her. It would mean resigning myself to a future that was far from what I hoped for her. It would mean accepting that her brothers would suffer through her illness. And I just couldn't.

Instead, I fought, until my fingers bled, and my eyes burned. I sought second, and third opinions, I frantically researched all night long. I fought until I had nothing left to uncover, and nothing left within me.

But what I didn't understand is the enormous difference between acceptance and resignation. Where I thought I was fighting against acceptance, I was really pushing back against resignation – states which are often confused.

Where resignation is a passive state of defeat, acceptance is an active response that leads to adaptation and growth.

Resignation feels like defeat. It's an overwhelming and disheartening emotion that can lead to a sense of hopelessness, a loss of control, and ultimately, emotional withdrawal. In resignation, there is a focus on what your child won't be able to do, and the limitations that lie ahead. This heavy sense of defeat can mean that parents feel there is nothing they can do to improve their child's life, or their own, which can lead to a deep sense of sadness and exhaustion. Parents experiencing resignation can often emotionally withdraw from those around them, turning away from connection to shield themselves from future pain and disappointment.

Acceptance, on the other hand, empowers parents to actively engage with their child's diagnosis: to seek understanding, to explore the best options, and to become a fierce advocate for their child's needs.

Does acceptance mean you need to feel good about the situation? Not at all. It's still hard and it's still sad. But it does allow parents to find a sense of hope for the future, even if that future is different from the one that they had originally envisioned. Even if that future is different to the future that lies ahead for their siblings or peers.

In the words of Desmond Tutu;
"Hope is being able to see that there is light despite all of the darkness."

Acceptance is a powerful word and a positive emotion that allows you to adapt to the challenges in your path. In acceptance you can establish new routines and discover new therapies. You can build a network of support around you and your family. Acceptance allows you to celebrate the wins and find joy in the achievements, even if they are small.

Acceptance is also one of the greatest gifts you can give your child and your entire family. When you understand your child's unique challenges and individual strengths, you can foster a deeper connection with them. Love stems from being seen, understood and valued for exactly who you are. When a family adapts to a difficult diagnosis it can open the door to long-term growth and a mindset of possibility, instead of the weight of impossibility.

For me, acceptance meant acknowledging the painful reality that the littlest love of our lives had a rare genetic disorder, and that this would become a massive part of our world. Once I understood that accepting my daughter's diagnosis was a state of empowerment, and that the future held possibility, the tsunami of rage dissipated. I wasn't being asked to accept the possible loss of her, I was being asked to accept that my life's purpose would involve fighting for her

- for her health, and her happiness and her future. I didn't need to accept the loss of her before we had even begun the fight. I'm not being asked to accept a life of pain and suffering for her, and in fact I refuse to accept that. Instead, I advocate for her, for alternatives, for new possibilities, for different treatments, to remove (or reduce) that pain. Much the same way that I advocate for my other children and help them move forward in their individual lives with strength, happiness and purpose.

Ultimately, acceptance is an adaptive, hopeful response that will help you find meaning and purpose, even within the challenges. Reaching acceptance however can be a gradual process and does not mean the removal of all pain and hardship, but it can provide a foundation of strength for you to move forward upon.

"In the midst of winter, I found there was, within me, an invincible summer. And that makes me happy. For it says that no matter how hard the world pushes against me, within me, there's something stronger – something better, pushing right back."

- Camus

Guilt - An Unwelcomed Extra

From the moment we conceive, our focus shifts, from caring solely for ourselves to caring for our child. We research and learn, we anticipate and prepare, we evolve, and we wait.

We carry our child in the very cells of our body, and we quietly promise to keep them safe. We dress-rehearse their lives, wondering who they will be, who they will become, and what awaits them. We make jokes about the flutters and kicks we feel, predicting future football players or dancers. We wonder whether our child will have our sense of humour or our partner's love of the water.

We imagine ourselves as loving parents, and we can almost feel their little arms around our neck, or the flutter of their eyelashes on our cheeks. Without realising it, we have mapped out a lifetime of possibilities for our little one, none of which include the diagnosis of a life-threatening condition.

Which is why, when your child is first diagnosed, immense feelings of loss and grief can often lead you to try to make sense of how something so devastating could happen. We need to apportion responsibility, to find someone or something to blame. The idea that there is no rhyme or reason to it, no one to blame, and nowhere to direct your pain, is unfathomable.

Without a direction for their pain, parents often turn inwards, asking themselves if they somehow made this happen, or what they could have done to prevent it. This interminable guilt just adds another layer to the heaviness of diagnosis, and it becomes heavier still when parents keep it to themselves – unable to hear the words out loud, or risk having their worst fears confirmed. Even if you share these fears with your medical team, there is often nothing a doctor can say to alleviate this sense of guilt. Such is the ferocity of those thoughts.

Like all emotions, guilt at a time of intense emotional turmoil can often appear unreasonable and won't make much sense to those around you, however it may comfort you to know that it's a silent pain that's being echoed in hospitals and homes all around the world. You are not alone.

It wasn't until we were deep into the world of oncology that I learned the most painful truth of all – that we're all carrying guilt, that it makes no sense to anyone but us, and that it will continue to bring us to our knees, even when we think we're done with it. We lug our guilt around with us as we carry our child from one specialist to the other, as we sit beside hospital beds, as we pray for stable tests or an uneventful appointment. We carry it like it's our burden to carry, like it's our responsibility to hold. Carefully, like a child.

I've spoken to parents who have bravely shared their greatest fear with me - that their child's diagnosis is their fault. Their reasons vary, from an existential sense of punishment for past wrongs, to the use of chemicals in the home. Some believe they chose the wrong house, with power lines too close, contaminated soil, or simply bad energy. Others feel it must have been their diet or a glass of champagne they had while pregnant. The reasons are as varied as the diagnoses, and none have any scientific basis.

Some parents can't articulate their guilt at all – only that it was their job to bring their child into the world safely, and they feel they have failed.

Sometimes parents berate themselves for not seeing the signs of their child's condition earlier, believing that if they had seen the signs, they could have somehow prevented it. Other times, particularly in the case of genetic conditions, parents fear they may have "passed on" the illness or exposed their child to an environmental factor which has triggered it.

While it's human nature to try to look for reasons, often there isn't one, and your guilt is an enormous burden that is deeply damaging. Dr. Shefali Tsabary, a clinical psychologist, often discusses parental guilt. She says;

"There is no greater burden on a parent
than the guilt of believing they were somehow responsible
for their child's struggles."

What this all speaks to is one beautiful, painful, truth – our love for our children is greater than anything else. It's innate. We are hardwired to love, nurture and protect our children, and in the shadow of that enormous love sits our grief, masquerading as guilt. We must try to make sense of how this could happen, and we feel it's our job to take responsibility for it.

However, it is not your fault that your child is sick. It is not your fault that your child has been diagnosed with this condition. Nothing you did has caused this, and nothing you could have done would have prevented it. You simply do not have that kind of power in this world.

Let me say that again.
This is not your fault.

In a world where uncertainty is almost obsolete, where access to information is always at our fingertips, it's difficult to accept that sometimes bad things just happen. Sometimes there is no explanation. And often we will never know why.

Sometimes, bad things just happen. And sometimes there's nothing we can do to stop them from happening.

If you're struggling to overcome feelings of guilt, please be gentle with yourself. Moving through guilt is a gradual process that involves self-compassion, strong supportive networks, and effective coping strategies.

This is one of those times when you'll find comfort and emotional relief in connecting with parents in similar situations, who will likely lean into your feelings with empathy, validation and practical advice. If you find these feelings are overwhelming you, seek help from a counsellor or psychologist, or speak to your hospital social worker.

A note for the quietly wounded,

Vulnerability. Is there a more powerful word to describe what it means to love?

Loving someone deeply will evoke a deep sense of vulnerability at one time or another.

Deeply loving someone you fear you could lose, without any guarantee of a future, requires you to be vulnerable on a whole other level.

Remaining open—and not shutting the door, or building barriers, or hiding away—requires significant courage.

But it also leaves space for gratitude, joy, and laughter.

Having a child with a complex or life-threatening medical condition is like living with an open wound. I cover it up, but sometimes it weeps, seeping through the layers until you can't help but see it.

Some people turn away for fear of having to acknowledge it. Some people turn towards it—with a kind word, a smile, or a new dressing for the wound.

I'm starting to understand that those who turn towards you have already learned this one powerful truth: that to be vulnerable is a strength, not a weakness.

It takes courage to wear my heart on my sleeve, to let my wound seep a little, to love my sweet girl so deeply—with no guarantee of a future. With all my heart. Infinitely.

Whatever you do, my friend, never stop being vulnerable. Your vulnerability makes you beautiful. Your bravery makes you shine. You are strength. You are power. You can do this.

Whatever it takes,
Me x

CHAPTER 5
Vulnerability Towards Courage

Nobody sits comfortably in vulnerability. To be vulnerable is to be exposed—to sit wide open to the possibility of harm or emotional pain. The word itself comes from the Latin vulnerare, meaning "to wound" or "to hurt," so it's no surprise that vulnerable in English is defined as "the quality or state of being exposed to the possibility of being attacked or harmed, either physically or emotionally."

To be vulnerable then is to be in a position where you may be either physically or emotionally wounded or hurt.

Could we also say that an appropriate definition would be, "to have a critically or chronically unwell child?"

Loving your child deeply and facing a future that feels uncertain and frightening leaves you susceptible to being wounded or hurt. To feel vulnerable during this time is almost inevitable. Your heart has been exposed, you're dependent upon medical professionals to make health decisions that are in the best interests of your child, and you're walking an unfamiliar and deeply uncertain path. I would hazard a guess that you have never been more vulnerable.

However, without vulnerability, there can be no courage. Without courage, there can be no growth.

Dr Brené Brown, a widely renowned vulnerability expert, speaks of vulnerability as being a measure of courage—of showing up with bravery even when there is no certainty around the outcome. We cannot become stronger, we cannot grow our resilience, we cannot hear the fierce roar in our pained hearts unless we acknowledge that we are vulnerable in this moment. When we deny our vulnerability, we deny our ability to grow and connect.

It makes me think of the time my little one told me she didn't like being called brave, because every time someone told her she was brave, something bad was about to happen. She was five years old, and she wasn't wrong. And yet, her exposure to being hurt or wounded has made her the most courageous and resilient person I know.

While vulnerability may feel painful and exposing, it allows us to grow as humans. Through vulnerability comes connection with others, and connection to the community in which you live. When you share your hurt and pain, it allows honest connections to be built with the people around you. In a sense, it gives permission to others to drop the mask of indifference and share their honest life experiences as well. This is why new friendships can be born, and old friendships deepened, in the darkest moments of life.

Further, speaking openly and vulnerably about difficult emotions can diminish their power, allowing you to process and move past the emotion or experience more easily.

There is no shortage of psychologists and thought leaders discussing vulnerability and its links to courage. However, when we refuse our own vulnerability and hold ourselves hostage to the idea that to share is a weakness, we allow our fears to grow out of proportion to the moment.

Psychologists speak of the importance of self-compassion in these moments—that being kind to oneself during moments of struggle is crucial for embracing vulnerability. This self-compassion helps individuals accept that it's okay not to have everything figured out, and it's okay to be imperfect. We are all imperfect, and we are all imperfectly showing up to life's more challenging moments.

When we look at vulnerability from the perspective of caring for a critically or chronically unwell child, vulnerability may show up as:

- Emotional exposure – experiencing a range of raw emotions, such as fear, anxiety, sadness, and helplessness, especially when witnessing your child in pain.
- Feeling uncertain – you may be facing a sense of powerlessness, in being unable protect your child or to control the progression or outcome of their illness.
- Needing support – having the courage to ask for help, or being open to receiving support from family, friends, healthcare professionals or support groups. Accepting help can be difficult for some people and can be tied up with unreasonable expectations of needing to do it all yourself. Sometimes you might perceive the acceptance of help as an admission that you are struggling. Being open to support, however, strengthens and deepens our connections with others and fosters a sense of community.
- Navigating shame – You may feel a sense of shame in being unable to handle everything yourself or feeling unable to

maintain optimism or hope in the face of the diagnosis. Often people with a high expectation of their own strength can feel a deep sense of shame as they experience the complexities of emotions that come with a traumatic situation.

- Courage in caregiving – it takes vulnerability (and strength) to continue to show up for your child - in caregiving, advocating, making medical decisions, and staying present with your child - despite the heavy emotional toll.
- Hoping - maintaining the courage to hope in the face of fear and uncertainty.
- Loss of identify – you may be struggling with your identity in the face of having a sick child. When your identity becomes tethered to the caregiving and advocacy of your child you tend to lose sight of yourself as an individual, and you put aside your own goals and needs.
- Allowing space for grief and acceptance – many parents suffer through grief for the loss of their child's health, the future you had planned for them, or just for the normalcy of their 'old' life. This grief is complex and multilayered and can be difficult to navigate without professional help.

Your child's diagnosis has thrust you into a world of intense emotions and uncertainty. While psychologists can encourage us to embrace our vulnerability, it's something that takes time and practice. Go gently with yourself. In time, your courage will lead to greater emotional resilience and deeper connections as you navigate this journey.

A note of solidarity for the ones who hurt,

There were days when the rage practically seeped from my pores. If it could have manifested itself, it would have been a field of charred remains. I was restless and angry beyond explanation. I couldn't sit still.

I listened to words being thrown around like confetti. Careless, kind, painful words.

"Everything will be alright." "She'll be fine." "You're strong." "You're right where you need to be right now."

But they were wrong.

Everything wasn't okay.

My baby wasn't okay.

I was broken.

This wasn't supposed to happen.

My close friends faced my fury with love and good humour. I had one friend who would have entire conversations with me where we just said 'Fuck'. A lot. Creatively. My closest friends bought me a pass to a smash pit.

I knew I felt so much more than anger, but I couldn't cope with all the other things I was too. Scared, let down, vulnerable, without hope. Despairing.

Anger felt like control and I had so little control left in my life.

It was only the inside of my car and the floor of the shower that saw the underbelly of my pain. It poured from my broken heart like the lyrics of an angry song. It spilled from me like poison. It tore at my flesh and pulled at my hair. It physically hurt - a desperate respite from the emotional pain.

My friend, it's okay to be angry and hurt. It's okay to be all the things. Just don't let the heat from the fire consume you.

This too shall pass.
Love, Me x

CHAPTER 6
Slow Hope

Hope allows us to imagine a brighter future, from a position of present pain.

Psychologically, hope draws on two essential capacities: the ability to envision a meaningful outcome, and the belief—however faint—that steps toward that outcome are possible and achievable.

Sometimes, such as in the case of having an unwell child, it can be difficult to hold onto hope amidst pain. Hoping for a better outcome can often feel pointless—or, worse still, dangerous—and when the act of hoping becomes too great, the end goal can feel unattainable.

However, without hope, we become inert; trapped in our grief and frozen in our trauma, no longer moving forward. When hope becomes lost to us, we move into a state of hopelessness and, ultimately, despair. And this, my friend, is when you need to find and hold onto hope the most.

The thing to remember is that hope can be small. It can be slow It can be gentle.

Hope doesn't need to roar in the night or front up with chest armour on. It doesn't need to be solid or predictable or driven. It isn't always written in neon signage. Instead, hope can be the whisper you barely hear, in a world that feels too loud. It can be a soft landing in a hard landscape. It can be the squeeze of a little hand, the gentle tucking in of blankets on a tiny bed, or a smile between tears.

Slow hope grows gently where certainty cannot. It's a seed planted in a broken field, feeding from a trickle of water.

Slow hope is the soft exhale between words of love and affirmation, and the gentle wish for a moment in time that is kinder, or easier or happier.

Slow hope is in the pause between words, and the whisper between heart and mind.

In the words of Emily Dickenson:

> *"'Hope' is the thing with feathers*
> *That perches in the soul—*
> *And sings the tune without the words—*
> *And never stops—at all—."*

Hope keeps us tethered to the possibility of a brighter future. Clinical studies and suicide risk assessments consistently find that hopelessness—more than depression or anxiety alone—is the strongest predictor of suicide risk. It's not the absence of suffering that matters —it's the belief, even faintly held, that the suffering might lessen, that tomorrow could look different, that there's still something or someone worth holding on for.

Dr Emily Musgrove, clinical psychologist and author, speaks beautifully about the importance of hope, and I encourage you to listen to her thoughts. She reiterates the point that without hope we are without a future. This was demonstrated in the work of psychiatrist Aaron Beck, whose Hopelessness Scale is still used today in clinical settings. Beck found that people who saw their problems as unchangeable and their pain as endless were at the highest risk of suicide. He found that it wasn't necessarily those who had the most severe symptoms of depression or anxiety that were most at risk of suicidal thoughts, but those who had lost sight of any meaningful future.

In this context it becomes critical that small acts of self-care are enacted, and that support is sought from whomever is best placed to deliver it—from friends, peers, family or professionals. By giving voice to the hopelessness within, we can dampen the threat response our body is experiencing, and begin to cultivate hope—slowly, gently, and with love.

Hope can often be confused with optimism, and many a well-meaning bystander will tell you to remain optimistic in the face of your child's diagnosis. However, the two are quite different. Where optimism is a simple wish that everything will work out in the end, hope is active and grounded. Hope is a cognitive belief that by undertaking certain actions, a better outcome awaits.

To paraphrase the words of N.T. Wright, a British theologian and author:

> *"Hope rolls up its sleeves and gets to work,*
> *while optimism sits back and watches."*

Finding Hope

In 1946, Viktor Frankl, a Holocaust survivor and psychiatrist, published his book 'Man's Search for Meaning', which was part memoir, part psychological reflection. In the book, Frankl recounted his traumatic experiences as a prisoner in Nazi concentration camps during World War II and introduced the world to his psychological reflections on hope. Frankl's book has sold millions of copies worldwide and continues to be deeply influential, especially for those seeking hope during suffering or grief.

Frankl theorised that hope can be found by discovering meaning in suffering, and in identifying ways to endure suffering while continuing to move forward. His approach, logotherapy (from the Latin word logos, which means 'meaning, reason or purpose'), teaches that while we can't always avoid pain, we can choose how we respond to it—and in that response, we can find purpose. His psychological theory centres on the idea that finding meaning in life—even in suffering—is what makes life worth living. This is sometimes referred to as 'tragic optimism,' where we embrace both the tragedy of life and the possibility of growth within it, without denying the pain or being blindly positive.

Frankl argued that our deepest motivation is not pleasure or power, but the search for meaning. He believed that even in the worst circumstances, like illness or loss, people can endure if they find a reason to keep going—through love, responsibility, or growth.

As the parents of an unwell child, this perspective can offer a quiet strength. The pain is real, but so is the meaning found in loving and caring deeply for your child, in showing up each day, and in choosing to hope even when the outcome is uncertain.

This is where slow hope becomes important. Slow hope is the ember of a flame within your heart. It's the tiny spark of light within your soul that encourages you to stay, to hold on, and to believe that within your pain, change is possible.

Slow hope allows you to set small goals. Those goals may be to put fresh sheets on the bed. Or to cook your favourite meal. They may be to see your child paint again, or to watch them turn the page of a book. They may include calling an old friend or seeking out that hug you desperately need. These small goals may feel insignificant, but each one gives you something more solid to stand upon. And with the setting of a goal, you're building the foundation for hope.

Slow hope doesn't come all at once—it drip-feeds gently into your heart, keeping the ember alive until it becomes a flame. As the flame grows, your goals may become bigger. Your goal may be for your child to participate in the sport they once loved, or for you to go back to work again. It may be to see your child reach their teenage years.

Sometimes you may need to recalibrate these goals as circumstances change, making them smaller or bigger as the situation dictates. And your resilient heart will find ways to do this—holding onto hope and finding meaning in the love and connection you have with your child.

CHAPTER 7
Navigating Relationships

The Impact on Your Marriage or Partnership

It's a well-known fact that partnerships that experience the ongoing or serious ill health of their child will experience increased relationship distress. In fact, research consistently shows that the parents of children with chronic or severe illnesses face a higher risk of divorce compared to parents of healthy children. Doesn't seem fair, does it?

The strain of an emotionally fraught situation can highlight existing cracks and exacerbate conflicts, tearing apart a union that may have been tenuous. Equally, relationships that had previously been happy and stable can find themselves on shaky ground during this time. That's because the pressure placed upon your relationship when you're confronted by the unexpected diagnosis or ill health of your child is unprecedented and significant.

You haven't done this before.

This is not the same old argument you've been having about unpacking the dishwasher.

This is next level.

This is pain and grief and worry, combined with lack of certainty, lack of sleep, and fear.

It's a turbo-charged situation, and you cannot underestimate the potential impact on your relationship. If you do one thing today, turn to each other and acknowledge that this is hard—that you may not always agree—and that you're in unknown territory. If you don't name it, you can't address it. So, first things first: get comfortable with vulnerability, and then try to safeguard your relationship before the cracks become craters. Before your resentment becomes too heavy to lug around with you (you know, on top of the guilt, fear and anger you're probably holding on to).

It's no surprise that research shows there is a direct correlation between the severity, duration and intensity of the child's illness (particularly as it impacts caregiving) and a higher risk of divorce or separation. The tougher the situation, the higher the level of marital strain.

This can feel disheartening—and even alarming—however, a relationship that navigates a difficult and emotional journey together can also be strengthened by the shared experience. Often, it's a matter of acknowledging the risk factors and scaffolding your relationship to withstand the storm. You may discover that together, you are stronger than the storm.

To better understand how relationships fall apart during times of intense stress, it's useful to consider factors such as emotional stress, financial pressure, caregiving imbalances, different coping styles, social isolation, anticipatory grief, and trauma. In this maelstrom of changed personal and family circumstances, so many forces come into play.

The emotional toll of facing your child's diagnosis and the challenges it brings can often lead to a sense of disconnect between you and your partner. An inability to communicate your fears and concerns can heighten conflict and reduce intimacy. What may appear to be apathy or indifference could actually be masking a deep and profound sense of fear and loss of control.

Having an unwell child can bring financial stresses to the forefront. Families often face the loss of an income when one partner becomes the primary caregiver. Add to this increased medical bills, hospital parking costs, and the price of therapies and interventions, and the pressure becomes enormous. This financial strain can feed into resentment—particularly if one partner is perceived to be living a semi-normal life by going to work and engaging in the outside world, while the other has assumed full-time caregiving duties.

There is often a lack of appreciation for the trauma the primary caregiver experiences: attending appointments, administering medications, and providing consistent emotional support, all while keeping the family functioning. The resulting imbalance can lead to resentment within the relationship. When compounded by a loss of personal identity and social isolation, the cracks in your partnership can deepen. These feelings may also be difficult for the working partner to fully accept, especially if they feel burdened by their role as financial provider.

Emotional distance can also grow when partners cope with the diagnosis differently. For example, one parent may become fixated on researching treatments and options, while the other avoids the topic altogether. One may be optimistic and dismiss the worries, or be unwilling to acknowledge how hard this truly is. This mismatch in coping can quietly erode the connection you share, just when you need it most.

If your child's condition is serious or potentially life-threatening, one or both of you may be experiencing anticipatory grief. Disconnection during this period can be devastating. While anticipatory grief is sometimes a way to emotionally prepare for loss, not everyone wants—or is ready—to face that possibility. You may also be grieving the future you imagined for your child, even if you can't yet put words to it.

Another under-recognised stressor is social isolation. You might lose touch with your old support systems, cut off by caregiving demands or the need to protect your child from infections. Suddenly, no more barbeques, drinks out, or play dates. Your world shrinks, and your partner becomes your only emotional outlet—despite the fact that you're also going through the same trauma. Additionally, many parents of critically ill children experience symptoms of post-traumatic stress, which can significantly alter relationship dynamics. It's a lot. Overwhelming, even. So, what can you do?

Put in place measures to protect your relationship. These are vital if you want to strengthen your bond through this experience.

And often, the most important measures are the ones that protect you. When you show up as your healthiest, most grounded self, you give your relationship the best chance of surviving and even thriving.

Effective communication is a powerful antidote to disconnection. Couples who maintain strong, open, and safe lines of communication are better equipped to cope. Yes, vulnerability is uncomfortable—but it also leads to deeper connections and greater emotional intimacy. This holds true to your romantic relationship just as it does for friendships and family bonds.

Leaning on your broader networks is crucial. (Other chapters in this book explore how to build and rely on your network). Your community might include peer support groups, hospital programs, or local organisations. Let them support you.

Counselling, if accessible, can be a valuable tool—for both individual and couple's work. While therapy may come with a cost, you'll find resources throughout this book to help you build resilience and manage overwhelm. Surround yourself with people who face life's challenges with courage and honesty. Avoid those that lean heavily into negativity. Friends who genuinely care about your wellbeing—and about your relationship—are gold.

Developing shared, mutually agreed coping strategies can prevent conflict and disconnection. Write these strategies down and display them somewhere visible as a regular reminder. You might include things like:
- Attending key medical appointments together
- Making joint decisions about treatment
- Committing to regular counselling
- Carving out quality time to reconnect
- Giving each other permission to take time out alone.

If possible, arrange for respite care—whether that's a trusted friend, family member, or formal provider—so that you and your partner can recharge and prevent burnout.

Whatever happens, remember: you're both hurting. You may not show it in the same way, but as the caregivers of an unwell child, you're both in pain. Showing up for one another with grace and assuming good intentions can shift the tone of your interactions. Caring for your partner's wellbeing as much as your own can be transformative—but only if it's mutual.

Conflict is not the enemy. Healthy, honest conflict can be a way forward. Don't be afraid to argue. Don't shy away from difficult conversations. Be open. Speak your truth. Sometimes clearing the air is exactly what you need to reconnect—and keep going, together.

Friendships During a Crisis

When life unfolds in unexpected ways or veers off course, it's natural to turn to the people closest to you to help weather the storm. There's an expectation that as the ground beneath you crumbles, your friends or family will stand with you in support—offering love, understanding, and a solid presence. A safe harbour in which to ride out the storm. But when the reaction you receive is one of silence, detachment, disbelief, or even dismissal, the weight of disappointment and hurt can be overwhelming. The silence that follows your plea for help can be deafening.

The truth is, most people will feel completely out of their depth when confronted with the diagnosis of your child. They may struggle to find the right words or the right ways to support you. A difficult diagnosis can bring up feelings of awkwardness, fear, or confusion for family and friends, and they may not know what to say. This uncertainty can result in conversations that feel insensitive, thoughtless, or uncomfortable.

Understanding why people behave or speak the way they do can be helpful in maintaining the relationships that may ultimately sustain you throughout this journey. That said, it's also worth recognising that some friendships may not survive this ordeal—and as painful as it is, sometimes it's for the best. It's okay to walk away from a friendship that no longer serves your wellbeing.

Over countless conversations with other parents walking similarly painful medical paths with their children, I've found that the responses of friends and extended family often fall into broad categories. I call these: the Diminishers, the Pessimists, the Optimists, the Avoiders, the Helpers and the Unicorns.

Please remember: as imperfect humans, we often shift between these categories when faced with trauma. This framework isn't intended to judge, but to help us better understand—and maybe find a little more grace—in an otherwise unfathomable situation.

The Diminishers

A Diminisher will often downplay the severity of the situation, and the pain or grief you're feeling. Without intentionally disrespecting you, they may call into question the diagnosis itself, or the proposed treatment plan. This can often have the unintended consequence of making you feel shame for the grief you're experiencing, leaving you to question the intensity and validity of your fears.

Diminishers may say things like:

- "At least it's not cancer."
- "80% survival is pretty good."
- "I know someone who went through exactly this and they're totally fine."
- "It could always be worse. At least it's not [insert another illness]."
- "Nobody knows what the future holds. I could be hit by a bus tomorrow."
- "Is that exactly what the doctor said?"
- "That seems unlikely to happen."

The Pessimist

A Pessimist will head straight to catastrophising the situation, speaking to you with a sense of worry and even inevitability. They tend to over emphasise the worst-case scenario, and express doubts about the chances of recovery. A well-intentioned Pessimist may attempt to connect with you in empathy and understanding, however, their fear for the future and the uncertainty of the diagnosis can negatively colour their support, leaving you feeling more stressed than supported. They will often place themselves in the picture and repeatedly reinforce that they couldn't imagine going through what you are going through.

A Pessimist may say things like:
- "I don't know how you do it. I couldn't cope if that was my child."
- "I wouldn't be able to get out of bed if that happened to me."
- "How are you so brave?"
- "I know someone who went through this, and their family fell to pieces."
- "I hope treatment works, but you hear so many stories like this that don't end well."

The Optimist

The Optimist, while well-meaning, will approach you with overly positive statements that can unintentionally downplay the gravity of the situation. Their comments are intended to be well-meaning and uplifting, but can often feel dismissive or invalidating, as they fail to acknowledge the emotional weight you're carrying.

The Optimist is often guilty of falling into the trap of using toxic positivity. In trying to approach you with hope, the Optimist can avoid discussing the very real fears or struggles you're facing, which can lead to a feeling of isolation.

The Optimist will often say things like:
- "Everything happens for a reason."
- "God wouldn't have given you this challenge if he didn't think you were strong enough to cope with it."
- "You are exactly where you're meant to be right now."
- "Everything is going to work out okay."

- "Everything will be okay in the end. If it's not okay, it's not the end."
- "Your child needs you to stay positive."
- "Just be grateful for what you have."

The Avoider

The Avoider may be the one who breaks your heart the most. It's the person you thought would be there for you in your time of need, only to discover they're unable to talk about the situation—or worse, they have vanished entirely.

The Avoider is often completely unable to cope with the difficult emotions of your child's illness and may have a fear of saying the wrong thing. They often validate their silence or absence by claiming that they are giving you space to process or heal, or not wanting to get in your way. However, their silence can feel incredibly painful and is deeply damaging to a relationship. The risk is that you, as the one in most need of support, will feel deserted and betrayed.

What the Avoider needs to understand is that their silence is not saying nothing. In fact, it's likely that the person in need of support hears their silence loudly, as saying, "I don't care enough to talk about this," or "The journey you're on isn't important to me," or "I think you're overreacting." Or worse.

Their silence feels like an excruciating statement that you are not worthy of their support, time, or compassion, and may make you question your relationship. And worse, yourself.

The Helper

The Helper is the doer and the organiser. They will actively seek out ways to support you and your child, channelling their reaction to the diagnosis into practical action. They might organise a meal roster amongst friends, offer to support siblings, or perform helpful chores.

The Helper needs to be doing something tangible to feel valued and to help ease your burden. However, The Helper often doesn't recognise when they are overstepping boundaries. In their need to be of help, they may fail to recognise your fatigue, exhaustion, and overwhelm, insisting that you tell them what they can do to help, and often making contact multiple times a day. They may place their need to be involved ahead of your own needs.

They may say things like "Just tell me what you need done and I'll organise it," or "I'm trying to help but you're not letting me."

The reality is that very often you won't know what you need, as you focus all your energies on holding yourself and your family together.

The Helper needs to be wary that they don't become intrusive or offer unsolicited advice, and that they don't become the unofficial spokesperson for the family without permission. It's also worth noting, that some (not all) Helpers are drawn to the drama of the situation and won't be a long-term support for you.

The Unicorn

The Unicorn is the ideal support person, but a quick word of caution in managing your expectations. Just as unicorns don't really exist, nor does the perfect person, who responds in the right way, interpreting your needs and understanding your emotions perfectly every time. Expecting our family and friends to assume the role of a Unicorn all the time is not only unfair, but it will lead to disappointment. That's not to say they can't try to be a Unicorn friend some of the time!

If a loved one is reading these words, or if they ask how they can best support you, here it is:

The Unicorn friend is someone who tries their best to offer a calm, consistent presence and is willing to listen—even when it's uncomfortable, even when it's hard. Even when it hurts. Trust me Unicorn: if it's hard for you, it's excruciating for your friend.

Finding the balance between leaving space for optimism while confronting the realities of the situation is no small thing. The Unicorn friend offers to help in a way that is most needed, like dropping siblings into the hospital, or prepacking sandwiches to freeze for their lunchboxes. This approach balances empathy with action in a way that feels considerate and empowering.

The Unicorn knows that small, simple statements of support, such as "I'm here for you," are worth their weight in gold and checks in with you with a quick message to see how things are going. They know that help is best offered in concrete ways, such as collecting kids from school, or doing a load of laundry, and they understand that you may be too overwhelmed to articulate those needs.

The Unicorn doesn't always know what to say and is comfortable acknowledging that. And so, they say, "I really don't know what to say," or "I'm sorry this is happening to you," or "The strength you're drawing on right now is enormous," or "I know it hurts, but you aren't alone."

The Pain of Unmet Needs

It's hard not to internalise your hurt when someone close to you lets you down, especially when your emotions are already raw and your heart already hurting. However, no one can be the perfect support all the time, and feeling disappointed in the way your family or friends are showing up for you is an almost inevitable part of the diagnosis journey.

The reality is, they don't know what you're going through, and they don't know what to say to you. You may not even know what you need in this time of emotional upheaval. However, often, you'll find that those who best understand and can offer the most support are those who have been through a difficult experience themselves.

Recognising the difference between those who are confused about how to support you, and those who have left you without any support, is vital. When you face the absence of support, it can be a painful lesson in recognising who truly stands by your side, and ultimately in letting go of relationships that are strong during times of ease, and absent in times of hardship. While this can add to your heartbreak, it can also be a moment of clarity, and an opportunity for growth. It allows you to reclaim your strength, reassess your needs, and hold tight to those friendships that nourish your battered soul.

The (Stupid) Things People Say

Sometimes people should just let a hug do all the talking, rather than get tangled up in comments that are unhelpful at best and damaging at worst.

For example:
- Reminding the parent of a critically ill child that they must be strong is wildly unnecessary. No one knows strength like a parent fighting for their child.
- Reminding you to 'take care of yourself', though well intentioned, is unhelpful. Your job right now is simply to continue. Surviving is the new thriving. You're holding the oxygen mask firmly to your child's face and sometimes drawing a little air from it yourself. Do not let self-care become one more thing you feel guilty about not doing well.
- While it may seem helpful, suggesting alternative therapies or recommending an infamous doctor in another country is fraught with risk. Medical parents are endlessly researching, reading and learning about their child's condition, on repeat. They already know. Suggesting they haven't done all they could do will haunt them forever. If you want to make a suggestion, ask first if they'd like to hear it.

Calmly and carefully setting boundaries for yourself may assist in gently warding off unhelpful comments, as well as dealing with the varied responses from friends. Being firm and clear, rather than angry or emotional, will always be more effective, however in the moment our emotions can feel unpredictable and untethered. Rather than smack someone in the head for suggesting you try Goji berries, preparing a few comeback lines to use in these situations is a safer idea.

For example:

- To the Pessimist - "I know you're trying to help, but this is really hard for us. It's a serious diagnosis, and we're doing our best to handle it."
- To the Optimist - "I appreciate you're trying to be positive, but we're just taking it one day at a time and are focusing on what's best for our child."
- To the Diminisher - "I understand that things could be worse, but this is the worst thing that's ever happened to us."
- To the Helper - "I can't think clearly enough to suggest what I need."
- To the Avoider - "When you say nothing, it makes me feel like you don't care."
- To the one who knows how to fix this - "Thank you for your suggestion, I'll look into Goji berries."
- To the suggestion that you need to be looking after yourself better – "My focus right now is on my child and our family. There'll be plenty of time for self-care later."
- To the one who reminds you to be strong or brave – "That's exactly what I'm doing."

Remember to show grace to yourself as well as others. It's okay to acknowledge that an imperfect or painful comment disappointed or hurt you. But trying to determine whether they're showing up as best they can (or not) will determine how you handle the relationship moving forward.

To the ones on the sideline,

It's not easy to be friends with someone going through childhood cancer, or any other significant life-altering illness or diagnosis. In fact, I think it's probably pretty damn hard. It's a one-sided friendship for a long time.

It's listening to the hardest of the hard, and the saddest of the sad. It's often not about laughter and good times, but about holding them in your arms while they cry. Or sitting in silence when they shut down.

It's swallowing your own fear that it could be your child, your baby, and wiping away the tears that spill from your eyes before they can see them.

It's messages, 'just checking in', and offering to care for their other children.

It's holding their sick child and willing them to get better.

It's a meal dropped at the door, sandwiches prepared and a chocolate cake, all ready for school lunchboxes.

It's asking the hard questions, even though it hurts, even though you don't want the answers, because all you want is to make it okay.

It's about saying, "this isn't okay" and "I love you. I see you. I have you".

It's looking grief in the eye and not looking away.

It's about being brave for the ones you love.

Their appreciation for you will know no bounds once they haul themselves onto the other side of this. You will have a friend for life.

Your friendship means everything.

Love, Me x

CHAPTER 8
A Chapter For Those Who Love You

Watching a loved one go through the trauma of having a critically or chronically unwell child can be heart-wrenching. It can be difficult to know what to do, what to say, or how to best support them. You may feel that nothing you do will make a difference, or that everything you're saying is landing wrong. You may not be able to cope with their anger or their tears of frustration and pain. You may not know how to help them navigate an unfamiliar world of hospital corridors, treatment protocols, and uncertainty. You may feel completely inept at comforting them, and completely unable to cope with the situation.

And that's okay. You don't need to be everything for them. But don't be nothing to them either. When you turn away from their pain, you're diminishing every terrible thing that's happening to them. And worse, your silence is loudly telling them that their experience does not matter to you. Your silence will make them question their own reactions, allowing shame to settle upon them, as they question whether they're overreacting, not strong enough, or simply unimportant. Don't fool yourself into believing that your silence isn't a weapon, and that it's not doing harm.

If I'm focusing heavily on this, it's for a simple reason - it's all too common for parents of unwell children to feel abandoned in their time of immense need. It's widely discussed in support groups, and in many instances can feel even more difficult than the medical issue at hand. The realisation that a parent does not have the support of their family or friends is a trauma in its own right.

So, what should you do?

All you need to do is show up. Lean in. Listen. Hug. Send a text. Be present. Be gentle. Be kind. Laugh when the mood strikes, listen when the mood is low. Hold their fear and grief in your hands as though it were the most precious thing on earth. Because it is.

Be the one who notices – has your loved one withdrawn from things that they previously enjoyed doing? Have they stopped answering the phone or responding to messages? Do you feel they've lost hope and could potentially be considering harming themselves?

Your friend, or your daughter, your son, your sibling, or your loved one is afraid. They are grieving. They're facing unimaginable pain and an enormous amount of uncertainty. Nothing is the same anymore. Ask them how they are. Simply ask. Or let them know you're thinking of them with no expectation of a reply.

It may sound counterintuitive, but asking your loved one what they need and expecting an answer is an additional weight upon their shoulders. They may not know. They're exhausted. They genuinely have no idea how to answer you. Please don't add guilt to their long list of difficult emotions, but instead try to think of what you might need if you were in their situation. It may be that there is nothing you can do that will make them feel adequate in the face of this trauma. But if you're genuinely seeking ways to help, start with practical offers – to pick up and drop off siblings, to prepare school lunch boxes, to drop off and pick up dry cleaning or washing. Just find something you think you could do and do it.

For more ideas on how to best provide support, refer to the previous chapter and be a Unicorn for the one you love. And if you're still not sure what to say, try these simple phrases:

- "How are you today?"
- "I'm in awe of your strength, but so sorry you need to be this strong."
- "I really don't know what to say."
- "I heard your child has (insert diagnosis). I'm so sorry, that must feel so hard."
- "I'm sorry this is happening to you."
- "I'll just drop a meal at your door and text you that it's there."
- "You must be finding it hard to keep on top of everything. Is it okay if I pop around to cut your lawn?"
- "I'm here if you want to talk. I'm also here to sit in silence. But either way, you're not alone."
- "It's just awful."
- "Would you like to talk about it?"
- "It's so hard to understand how something like this can happen."
- "Please don't feel you need to respond; I just want you to know I'm here."

Comfort In, Dump Out (The Circle of Support)

The Circle of Support can be a useful guide as to how to offer support to a loved one during a time of crisis. The concept was developed by clinical psychologist Susan Silk and her colleague Barry Goldman, who saw a need for a psychological model that allowed individuals to provide appropriate and helpful comfort during a time of crisis, based on proximity to the person at the centre of the crisis.

The model revolves around four simple words – comfort in, dump out. The Circle of Support visually depicts how to offer support in a time of crisis, such as divorce, death, illness or loss of any kind. The basic idea is that people in crisis sit in the centre of a series of social rings, like the rings on an archery board. The people in the outer rings offer support inwards, while sharing their emotions outwards.
Example:

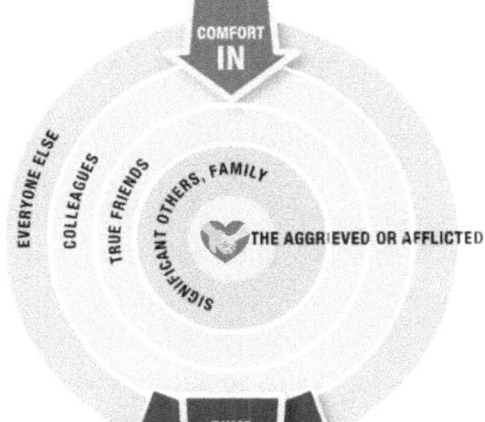

[3] https://abeautifulvoice.org/2020/01/06/how-to-unwrap-the-the-ring-theory-when-its-not-about-you/

When a child is unwell, that child sits at the centre of the ring. Depending on the age of the child, parents and siblings may sit in the closest ring to the centre, or they may be in the centre as well. For example, you can imagine a teen holding their own space in the centre, while a baby or younger child would have their parents in the centre with them.

The grief and emotional well-being of those in the centre of the model, and in the closest ring, becomes the focus of support. They are allowed to grieve, cry and worry as much as they need to, to all who surround them.

The next ring outwards might hold immediate family members, such as grandparents, aunts and uncles, as well as close friends who are intimately connected to the parents and child. The next ring from there might be other friends and work colleagues, and so on.

The further the rings are from the centre, the less affected they are by the crisis. Not unaffected—just less affected.

The job of those in the closest rings is a difficult one. While feeling all the emotions themselves, their role is to offer love, empathy and support inwards, while not burdening those in the centre of the circle with their own fears, emotions or concerns. This can be enormously difficult for some people, and they can be left with a sense of being excluded from the crisis, while also suffering emotionally themselves. This is where the following rings become important—to provide them with support and an outlet for their pain as well.

The rule of thumb is that everyone can offer comfort inwards, but they must only express negative emotions outwards. Venting inwards can add to the grief and emotional strain of those most closely impacted and can be extremely unhelpful. People outside of the centre who need to verbalise their worries should seek support from the outside rings, or from their own social networks, rather than turning to those in the centre of the crisis.

If it feels as though you're carrying the weight of everyone's emotions and worries when you can barely carry your own, this model is for you. If you're able to share this with your loved ones, fabulous, but if not, ask someone you trust to have the discussion for you. Ideally, this would be someone who can talk it through with compassion and kindness, lifting the weight from your weary shoulders.

Continue to Love Their Child
(even when nothing is the same)

Sometimes children with particular diagnoses or who are going through specific treatments can look different to how they previously looked, in a way that's confronting for loved ones. It's important that you don't retreat or pull away from the family to protect your own feelings.

I know it's hard, and I know it's sad, but turning towards their visible pain instead of away from it is healing for all. If you can, ignore the feeding tube, the weight loss or gain, the muscle wasting, or the hair loss, and focus on playing a game with the child, painting a picture, kicking a ball, having a conversation, or doing a dance. Whatever it is the child loves, do that with them. Be that for them. Their parents will always remember your kindness. But if you can't do that, please don't put yourself in that situation. Their happiness if not at the expense of yours, and it's okay to know your limitations. Instead, try to offer support in other more comfortable ways, such as with a meal, a text message, a phone call or a card.

What Not To Do

The fact that you're reading this with the purpose of providing meaningful support means that you are already kicking goals. You've done the most important thing of all and have shown up with the intent to help. So, I want to tread gently here when I talk about what not to do and acknowledge that in most cases, people who participate in any of these behaviours don't do so with the intention to wound. And yet… if someone accidentally runs over your foot and says sorry, you're still hobbling around with a broken foot. Which is to say, that pain, intentional or otherwise, is still pain.

So, with that in mind, please avoid:

Doing nothing – As previously discussed, silence is enormously damaging, as is disappearing from your friend's or loved one's life. Please don't desert them in their time of need. Even if you have nothing to say, your presence says that you care.

Belittling their experience – Comparing their experiences to others who you perceive to be 'worse off' isn't comforting, it's diminishing the pain they're experiencing. Every situation is unique – every diagnosis, prognosis, complicating factor, treatment plan, side effect and emotional response differs from child to child and family to family.

Questioning their medical team – Unless you have valid and significant reasons to feel concerned that the child's diagnosis or means of treatment is incorrect, do not pretend to know more than the specialists do. It only adds an additional layer of worry upon the parents. If your concern is real, please encourage the parents to escalate the issue within the hospital system.

Shaming them – Their emotional response to the situation is real. Your opinion regarding the scale of that response is unnecessary. Until you have sat in a room and been delivered unthinkable news, do not presume to understand what they are feeling. It's not kind to tell them they are overreacting. It's not kind to question the seriousness of the diagnosis. It is not kind to tell them they need to get over it and/or move on.

Telling them this is part of God's plan – Or some variation of the theme that they're exactly where they need to be in the universe right now. Just no. A child is sick, a family is hurting. Being told it's all part of the plan isn't helpful right now. Maybe one day the family will have a different emotional response to this kind of sentiment, with time and hindsight, but not now. It's way too soon.

Starting a go-fund me or fundraising drive without their permission. This is a tricky one. Some families need this kind of support and will be enormously grateful, but it's always better to ask. For some, it will allow them to put work on hold while they focus on the immediate period following diagnosis. But for others, raising money may feel difficult or awkward, and they may not be enthusiastic about the idea. It's a very personal preference. For us, we weren't keen on a go-fund me and so a friend came up with the beautiful idea to make over our children's bedrooms. This felt like a win for all – those who really wanted to help could, our children were spoiled with something special, and there was no exchange of monies.

Overstepping - Sharing information that the family haven't yet shared, running charity events in the name of the child, or using unauthorised images of the child to garner sympathy or funds. This may sound appalling; however, you'd be surprised how many families have been deeply hurt and emotionally exposed by this kind of behaviour. Some people are drawn to a crisis and the attention it brings them by proximity.

Saying things that are likely to upset the parents – especially in the early days of diagnosis.

For example, please do not repeat the following:
- "How sad that it's your only *girl* who has the brain tumour."
- "Did you vaccinate your child?"
- "Did your child eat a lot of sugar?"
- "Maybe you'd just be better to let her go. What kind of a life will she have?"
- "Wow, you guys are so unlucky" and, a related question, "Who did you kill in your last life?"
- "Poor thing, she got hit with the unlucky stick, didn't she?"
- "Time to be a big girl."
- "You're really upsetting us all – it would be better if you didn't talk about it."

- "It doesn't look like you're looking after yourself."
- "I wouldn't be able to get out of bed if I were you."
- "It's just a benign brain tumour, isn't it?"

And so on. While some of these comments and questions may sound ridiculous, they are all things my husband and I have personally heard and walked away from.

To the one who's world has changed,

A few weeks after she began chemo, her hair began to fall out. She cried in pain as each follicle relinquished its hold, and I cried in pain as I felt life as we knew it slipping through my fingers.

I didn't know how painful it would be for her. No one warned me that she would scream if I stroked her hair. No one told me how it would feel to collect her beautiful hair from her pillow each morning, hiding it from her, from her brothers, from myself.

No one warned me of the pain of seeing her big brother, so little himself, cry as he held up a fistful of her hair, after simply stroking her head.

I threw it in the bin like it was nothing. But it was everything. It was the beginning.

Taking her out into the world after that was challenging. There is no more powerful visual than that of a child—or an adult—without hair. My life, my pain, was on display for the world to see.

My grief was hung around my neck like a neon sign.

Without knowing the details, everyone assumed they knew the story of my life. She had lost her hair, and I had lost my mask.

I found myself walking out of shops empty-handed after comforting a crying stranger or on the verge of tears myself. The sheer kindness, as well as the painful curiosity of the world around me, often brought me undone. I didn't know what to say, and so it became easier to just stay home. Home—where I couldn't see our sadness reflected in the eyes of strangers. Where the contrast between healthy and fragile wasn't as blindingly stark.

Home, where I could watch her twirl in her frothy tutus, dancing her way through life as though it were nothing at all. "No hair, don't care," we used to laugh. And, eventually, we meant it.

With love,
Me x

CHAPTER 9
Cultivating Calm

It may come as no shock to you that shoving down fear and grief and plastering on a smile doesn't lead to happiness. It leads to burnout. And burnout is a terrible place to be; it's where your body lets you down and your threshold for stress is so low you keep bumping your head on it. And when I talk about burnout, I'm talking about it in a medical sense, not as a fleeting emotion or an especially tiring week.

Burnout is a prolonged response to chronic stress. Recently the World Health Organisation changed its definition of burnout, calling it "a syndrome conceptualised as resulting from chronic workplace stress that has not been successfully managed." And make no mistake, when you have a chronically or critically unwell child, caring for them becomes your job.

When we experience trauma or profound stress, our body and brain go into survival mode. In the moment, we experience a surge of stress hormones, our heart rate increases, our breathing quickens, our muscles tense, and our digestion slows. If the stress is ongoing, cortisol will begin to suppress functions that are not considered essential for survival, such as immune function. If the stress becomes long term (days to months), the body's responses become stuck in an overactive state, leading to high blood pressure, a weakened immune system and hormonal imbalances. Before you know it, your sleep will be disturbed, your memory foggy, and you may begin to struggle with anxiety and depression.

Chronic stress can also interfere with deep, diaphragmatic breathing, which typically calms the nervous system. Stress tends to cause shallow chest breathing that bypasses the diaphragm, which can further amplify feelings of anxiety and create a feedback loop of stress and breathlessness. Shallow breathing can make you feel a sense of tightness in your chest and tension in your shoulders and may give you the feeling of being starved of air.

The vagus nerve acts as the body's communication highway between the brain and key organs, such as the heart, lungs and digestive system. Persistent stress can result in the vagus nerve struggling to work effectively, placing the body in a constant state of 'fight or flight' and weakening the body's ability to 'rest and digest.'

It's important to understand that trauma isn't just a memory – it's an experience stored within your body. The body and mind must work together to reestablish balance and regain a sense of safety and control, keeping burnout at bay.

How to Process Trauma

There are many well-known methods of processing trauma and stress within the body; however, sometimes it can be difficult to know where to begin or how to practice the right way. Let me just say, there is no right way. A few moments a day spent listening to your mind and body, to calming your nervous system, and reminding yourself to practice kindness and compassion is far better than beginning and ending your day with a clenched jaw and tight chest. Simply begin and see what happens.

Breathe

Practicing diaphragmatic or belly breathing is a well-known, research-based technique that counters shallow breathing and calms the body. It works by engaging the parasympathetic nervous system, which slows the heart rate, and promotes relaxation.

Some helpful breathing exercises include:

1. Belly Breathing - Place one hand on your chest and the other on your belly. Slowly inhale through your nose so that your belly rises, keeping your chest as still as possible. Exhale through your mouth, feeling your belly fall. Aim to breathe in and exhale for 4 to 5 seconds each.

2. Box Breathing - Breathe in for 4 seconds, hold for 4 seconds and exhale for 4 seconds. This cycle can be repeated for several minutes until you feel you have control of your breathing. You should feel refocused and have somewhat calmed the mind. Some people prefer to exhale for a longer period than the in-breath. Find what works for you.

3. Lion's Breath – This is an energizing breathing technique that has its origins in yoga. It can also help relax your jaw muscles. First, sit comfortably and spread your fingers out on your knees. Take a deep breath through your nose, then open your mouth and stick out your tongue (as far as it will go) as you exhale. Make a long 'haaaaa' sound as you exhale and try to look at the tip of your nose. Do this exercise 2 or 3 times in a row.

4. Humming Bee – This exercise requires you to be in a place where you can feel free to make a humming noise. To practise

the humming bee, sit comfortably and close your eyes. Relax your face and place your first fingers on the cartilage that partly covers your ear (as though you're about to block your ears with your fingers). Inhale gently and press your fingers into the cartilage as you exhale. Keeping your mouth closed, make a loud humming sound. Continue for as long as you want to. This technique also originates from yoga and focuses on creating a sense of calm and easing the muscles in your forehead. Research indicates this exercise is particularly good at reducing your heart rate, easing feelings of anxiety, anger and frustration.

Activating the Vagus Nerve

When we activate the vagus nerve, it allows the body to switch into a state of relaxation and recovery, slowing your heart rate, lowering blood pressure, and promoting deep and steady breathing. This works to reduce the stress and anxiety in your body, as well as aiding digestion. A well-functioning vagus nerve will also reduce the level of inflammation in your body and support a stronger immune system.

Methods of activating the vagus nerve include:
1. Deep breathing exercises, as above.
2. Humming, singing and chanting – stimulates the muscles around the vocal cords, which are connected to the vagus nerve.
3. Exposing your body to cold – splashing cold water on your face, taking a cold shower, or swimming in a cold body of water.
4. Meditation and mindfulness to promote stress resilience and deep relaxation.
5. Yoga and Tai Chi.

6. Gut health – the vagus nerve has a direct connection to the gut, so maintaining a good gut microbiome can greatly assist in managing overall wellness and resilience to stressful periods.

Affirmations

An affirmation is a short, positive statement that shifts your mindset and reaffirms feelings of power and hope. Some people find affirmations to be a positive and empowering way to stay grounded and hopeful through difficult times. You may choose to state your affirmation aloud each day, to internally focus on it through moments of challenge, or to write it down. Some people find a single affirmation, and it becomes their mantra of hope, and others cycle through them as a continual reminder of hope and courage.

Some examples of affirmations you might connect with include:
- "It's okay to feel what I'm feeling. I can handle this."
- "This journey is hard, but I can do hard things."
- "I am doing the best I can for my child, and that is enough."
- "It's okay to ask for help. I am not alone."
- "Together we will overcome these challenges."
- "Even in hard times I will find moments of joy."
- "I've faced hard times before, and I can do it again."
- "I have survived every difficult thing that's ever happened to me."
- "I trust that I will adapt and find solutions for my child's needs."
- "I deserve to look after myself, so I can look after my child."
- "I am here, I am important, I am supported."

- "I am strong and can get through this."
- "My child is unique and wonderful and loved, just as they are."
- "I am a source of love, hope and strength for my family."
- "This is a hard moment, but I will get through it."
- "I am loved, I am supported, I am going to be okay."

You can make up your own affirmation based on your feelings in this moment. For example, "Today I am (strong/hopeful/courageous), and I can handle (this test/this treatment/this diagnosis/this difficult moment)."

Journaling

If the idea of capturing your emotions and documenting your thoughts on paper appeals to you, journaling can be a powerful way of processing trauma and making sense of difficult experiences.

Journaling can assist in releasing stress and bottled-up emotions, which have been shown to improve mood and even enhance immune function. It's also a useful way to document events, which may be of interest to you in the future.

Some ideas to kickstart your journaling include:
- What were my first thoughts and feelings when I received the diagnosis?
- How am I feeling today?
- How has this experience changed the way I see life?
- What strengths have I discovered in myself?

- If I were to tell my story as one of resilience, how would it sound?
- What are my child's strengths?
- What hopes do I hold for my child's future?
- Three things I'm grateful for today.
- Three things that have been hardest today.
- Who has been a strong support for me?
- What has surprised me most by this experience?
-

You may also like to set some goals for your family, your child, or yourself, or some for well-being or physical goals to document and work towards.

Progressive Muscle Relaxation (PMR)

PMR involves tensing and releasing each muscle group, starting from your toes and moving to the tip of your head. The technique helps release physical tension associated with stress and creates a sense of bodily calm.

To do it properly, you need to lie somewhere comfortable, such as a bed. Moving progressively up your body, from your toes to your scalp, to the tips of your fingers, tense and name each body part. Hold that tension until your entire body is taut before reversing the process and relaxing each part of the body from head to toe.

One final burst of energy expenditure and relaxation for each of the muscle groups in your body is a surprisingly effective technique to encourage sleep and relaxation.

Body Scans

Gently and without judgement, mentally scan your body from head to toe, observing sensations of tension without trying to change them. This process is useful in promoting focus and awareness of the stress your body is holding.

While PMR is a more active approach to obtaining relaxation, body scanning focuses on mindfulness and acceptance and allows the mind to redirect away from anxious thoughts. There is no end goal or fix with a body scan, simply a gentle check-in with your body and an awareness of the tension it's holding.

Physical Exercise

Physical exercise is an acknowledged and recommended approach to combating stress. It's widely known that when you move your body, your brain releases endorphins or 'feel-good hormones,' which help alleviate feelings of stress and anxiety, lower cortisol levels, and improve sleep quality.

However, finding the time and space to exercise when you are in a period of crisis can feel almost impossible. Be gentle with yourself, and move as you can, and when you can. You may find that during periods of intense stress, you don't have the same stamina you may have had, and any exercise you do undertake can release pent-up emotions, resulting in floods of tears. You may also find it's just what you need to physically expel the stress of the day.

Tapping Into Your Creative Energy

Creativity is a beautiful way to tap into your emotions and process difficult feelings. Creativity can take the form of music, art, crafting, and dance, and is limited only by your imagination. Some people find it useful to keep busy when their child is in hospital, using the time to knit, journal or create a scrapbook of memories. Others find a joint project with their child can turn a difficult time into a treasured memory. Don't be deterred if creativity isn't your usual strength—just go with the flow and see where it takes you.

Emergency Measures

Sometimes we find ourselves in an acute moment of stress. This may occur when receiving difficult or bad news, when you're waiting for test results, or after a particularly difficult day or night. I've suffered what I think of as an instant migraine when hearing bad news and would begin to pre-empt and dread the physical symptoms of dysregulation that accompanied those days.

Should you find yourself needing quick emergency measures to disrupt anxious thought cycles and ground yourself in the present moment, try the following:

- Practise the 3-3-3 method. Without anyone realising, you can shift your focus from anxious thoughts to an immediate sensory experience, which helps to regulate the mind and body. To practise this technique, identify 3 things you can see, 3 things you can hear, and 3 parts of your body to move. This practice is widely recommended by mental health professionals to redirect focus and calm the nervous system.
- Squeeze your toes in your shoes. Squishing or curling your toes

in your shoes is a small progressive muscle relaxation (PMR) technique that allows you to focus on a physical sensation and can promote a sense of calm. Tensing your toes and then releasing them can reduce muscle tension and slow your heart rate.

- Practise slow and steady breathing. Calm, deep, measured breathing can be done subtly and can assist in slowing your heart rate and reducing blood pressure, allowing you to better cope in the moment.
- Repeating a self-compassion statement in your mind, such as "this feeling is temporary," or "I can handle this," or "this too shall pass." These can create a sense of inner reassurance and promote resilience.
- Visualise a space that's safe, secure, and happy. When my daughter was having her central line accessed for chemo, we would talk about the space we were visualising. Mine would always involve the beach, and hers often involved ice cream! I would sing the Daniel Tiger song to her: "Close your eyes and think of something happy."

To the one who's doing what needs to be done,

We talk a lot about bravery in our world— about finding small moments of bravery to get through the hardest of times. Step by step, moment by moment.

Bravery is often found in facing what lies ahead... the pain, the sickness, the fatigue and the grief... and doing it anyway, because sometimes there's no choice.

But what about the bravery in not knowing what lies ahead? In moving forward, in endless uncertainty, day after day.

For a time, every day, my little girl would ask me, "Mummy, after the dark and in the morning, what are we doing today?"

And then she would wait.

She'd wait for me to tell her if it was going to be a hospital day, or a treatment day— after the dark had gone and the sun had risen. She wanted to feel prepared. My poor, brave little soul.

Her lack of understanding, and complete powerlessness over the situation meant that she couldn't predict what was coming— today, tomorrow, and all the tomorrows. And if she couldn't see it coming, how would she know when to be brave?

And so, she was always primed for bravery. Little fists raised to an invisible enemy, waiting for Mummy to tell her when to fight.

And fight we did, fists raised together, asking fear to step aside, so we could do what had to be done.

Whatever it takes,
Me x

CHAPTER 10
Fear & Loss

Loss

In the Western world, we often struggle to speak of death. When amidst a medical journey, our language is often determined and action-driven. We fight, as though we can avoid or prevent the end of life, and we talk in terms of losing when death inevitably arrives. How many times have we heard variations of the phrase, "She fought so hard, but lost the fight"?

After the fight, we often soften our language to make it more bearable, using the gentler word 'lost' in place of the blunter option, 'died.' The concept of loss suggests the possibility of being found again, as though the one you miss is absent rather than truly gone. It also embodies the sense of loss that occurs within yourself, as you navigate the unfamiliar territory of grief. It aligns with the search for peace that follows the loss of a loved one, and the search for meaning and identity in your new world. So much has been lost.

When the natural order of parents aging and dying ahead of their children is threatened, and we fear losing our child first, it can be deeply distressing and challenging. We are biologically hardwired to protect our children, and a diagnosis forces us to confront the limits of our capacity to protect them from harm and ensure their well-being.

Fearing the death of your child following diagnosis is connected to a deep sense of loss of certainty. It's primal, paralysing and deeply painful. Within Western culture, we have become so used to certainty in our lives, easily accessing information and answers at the touch of a button—that we are unprepared for the sudden sense of fear and uncertainty that a diagnosis brings. The future and all its plans are no longer certain. We no longer know what tomorrow may bring. We are unfit for uncertainty. We cannot ask Siri to make it make sense for us, and we can't log onto a website and look for an expected forecast of the stormy times ahead. We can only move forward in uncertainty.

Anticipatory Loss

Fearing the loss of your child, or the loss of the future you expected for your child, is known as anticipatory loss. It occurs when something meaningful is coming to an end, and we begin grieving before the loss is fully realised. Anticipatory loss plays the important role of giving your heart and mind time to process the reality of change before it fully unfolds. Unlike sudden loss, anticipatory loss unfolds gradually, allowing you to make small steps towards adjustment.

Anticipatory loss explains the complex grief you may experience when you consider your child's future. You may find yourself grieving the loss of innocence for your child, of a life untouched by illness. You may grieve the childhood you expected for them, their diagnosis disrupting not only their experience of life, but also your family life. You may be grieving a loss of certainty for the future—for plans that may now never happen—for travel, or education, or life experiences. The losses you feel will be unique to your personal situation and may ebb and flow in intensity.

Anticipatory loss allows you to emotionally prepare for the challenges that lie ahead. When experiencing anticipatory loss, some days will feel far heavier and more difficult than others, and you may feel you're living with an emotional duality that can be exhausting—holding hope and fear in equal measures within your heart.

Dress Rehearsing Loss

Dress rehearsing loss is a psychological concept whereby you mentally prepare for loss by imagining it happening before it actually does. The brain tries to anticipate and control the emotional impact of grief. This can be both a coping mechanism and a source of anxiety. Dress rehearsing loss stems from a deep-seated love, where you may feel the need to practice losing your child, so that if it happens it doesn't come as such a shock. Many parents feel that if they don't prepare for the enormity of this loss that the loss itself—when it happens—will be unbearable. This is even true when the diagnosis itself is not life threatening.

Imagining your child dying is a deeply human response combining evolutionary survival mechanisms with intense emotional vulnerability. Your brain is perceiving a direct and serious threat to something precious to you and is hardwired to plan for and anticipate this danger. When you add to that the fear that arises from uncertainty, and a need to protect yourself from being blindsided by catastrophe, it becomes understandable that you begin to dress rehearse loss—to know how you might cope with such an event. I've spoken to loving parents who have planned what songs they would play at their child's funeral, then felt an enormous sense of shame in these thoughts.

How to Overcome Your Fears

Coping with loss—actual, anticipatory, or dress rehearsal—requires both emotional and practical strategies. Because your fear is rooted in love and connection to your child, the goal isn't to eliminate it, but to manage it in a way that allows you to still live meaningfully in the present.

It's important that you recognise anticipatory and dress rehearsal loss as real, and that you give yourself permission to grieve all you have lost and all that you fear losing. Take time to truly honour those feelings rather than brushing them aside. Instead of suppressing your emotions, recognise them as valid and give voice to them. It's well known that fear thrives on isolation, and by bringing our fears out and into the light we can help acknowledge and process them—diminishing some of their potency. Speaking to someone you trust about your fears can often provide clarity and can activate our brain to problem-solve, allowing us to brainstorm coping mechanisms rather than sitting in our anxiety. It also allows us to release the emotions that are feeding the fears, further de-escalating their power over us.

Grounding yourself in the present day or moment can be an effective way to avoid being pulled into an imagined future of pain. Remaining in the 'right now' through mindfulness exercises can help you appreciate the moment you are in. Deep breathing, deliberately noticing small details, and intentionally being present are all effective mindfulness tools. Ask yourself, "What is true in this moment?", breaking the cycle of anticipatory loss and future anxiety.

When you feel yourself catastrophising, it can help to reframe your thoughts. For example:

- "Right now I'm here with my child, and we're getting through this together."
- "This illness is hard, but we have the best medical support, and my child is strong."
- "I feel like this because I love my child."
- "It's okay to feel like this, but it doesn't mean that the worst will happen."

While anticipating loss may feel like a way to prepare for the future, it often steals the joy of the present. The best way to 'prepare' for loss is to fully embrace the time you have—making memories that will bring comfort if the much-feared loss arrives.

Find Professional Support

Therapy can be a powerful tool for navigating the overwhelming emotions that often accompany a child's illness. However, accessing professional support is a privilege—not everyone has the financial means or logistical access to engage in therapy, making it an unavailable option for many families.

If you do seek out professional support, therapists will often use Cognitive Behaviour Therapy (CBT) to help you identify catastrophic thinking, and help you reframe these thoughts. It can also be useful in teaching you thought-stopping techniques, which allow you to consciously stop yourself when you identify fearful or catastrophic thinking.

Another successful therapeutic approach is Eye Movement Desensitization and Reprocessing (EMDR), which addresses specific traumatic memories and allows the brain to process the complex emotions that accompany them. For many parents, the moment of diagnosis is a particularly emotional and multifaceted, and EMDR can help ease the impact. Many psychologists are qualified in both CBT and EMDR therapies.

Professional support, however, doesn't have to be in-person sessions with a psychologist. Not only can that be prohibitively expensive, but it can also be difficult to find the right practitioner, and waitlists are often ong.

If seeing a psychologist isn't an option for you, seek out supports or reputable information available through social media, or lean on friends who are therapeutic by nature. You know—the friend who is happy to share psychology memes, to talk about emotional topics, and embraces the frailty of the human experience. Or, follow psychologists online, listen to their podcasts, and absorb whichever pieces of wisdom resonate with you in that moment.

There are also online counselling services, which are often more affordable, as well as phone counselling available through charities.

A note for the one who stayed soft so their child could feel safe,

Imagine if you refused to succumb to anger and bitterness. If you let your pain and hurt slide gently into your soul, to sit softly, instead of throwing it outward, as others do, to hurt.

What if you learned to recognise the anger or meanness of those around you for what it is? Pain. Pure and simple.

Imagine how much kinder life could be if we all did that.

Imagine if you had the strength to reach into your pain and release it to the breeze—softening your heart, releasing your rage. Imagine how much safer the world would feel. For everyone.

You're going to feel it all throughout this journey. People will say things that hurt. People will do things that steal your breath away. Life will come at you.

Soften into it. Release the hurt. Don't hold onto the pain.

Remember that the small, gentle silences leave space for beautiful things to happen.

With love,
Me x

CHAPTER 11
Turning to Spirituality

Spirituality is a deep and personal way of connecting with something larger than ourselves—whether that's seen as God, the universe, nature, love, or simply the mystery of being alive. It's about seeking meaning and finding a sense of belonging beyond the physical world. Spirituality often helps people grapple with the big questions in life: Who are we? What is our purpose? What happens when we die? And in moments of profound grief, it's about holding onto hope when life feels unbearably heavy.

For many parents walking through the heartbreak of a child's illness, spirituality can become a quiet anchor—a way to hold onto a thread of connection and to believe that love is limitless, and doesn't simply end. It shows itself as prayers whispered, with hands clasped tight. It can be found in the signs that become a symbol for hope—a feather on the doorstep, a bird on the windowsill, or the repetition of numbers. Spirituality can show up in connectedness with others—in the kindness of the community that surround you, in the tears of those feeling your pain, or in the search for meaning amid chaos and suffering.

For some, spirituality can be found in meditation and quiet acts of reflection. For others, it is deeply rooted in religions lessons and practices. At its heart, it is a belief that there is more to life than this moment, and that there is a purpose behind our suffering. It whispers gently that even here, in the hardest of times, love matters most.

In looking for answers to the question of spirituality, I was reminded that people all over the world are walking this painful path alongside us—that they too have reached into the dark and whispered the names of their children into the still of the night. They have turned to different religions and philosophies to make sense of their pain.

In East Asian religions, I learned of Guan Yin, a being who has attained enlightenment but who chooses to remain in the world to help others. In compassion and mercy, she is said to hear the cries of the world and is depicted with a thousand arms and a thousand eyes—so she may see and comfort all who suffer. A mother-spirit who listens without turning away. It brings me peace to imagine her sitting quietly beside us, bearing witness to every beeping monitor and restless sigh.

In Christianity, I thought of the spiritual poem, Footprints in the Sand, written by Mary Stevenson. In the poem, a person dreams they are walking along a deserted beach with God, with two sets of footprints visible in the sand—one belonging to them, and the other to God. During a particular time of darkness and pain the person notices that only one set of footprints remains and asks God why He abandoned them during their time of grief. God responds:

> *"My precious child, I love you and would never leave you. During your times of trial and suffering—when you saw only one set of footprints—it was then that I carried you."*

The poem resonates deeply with those walking through pain. It reminds us that even when we feel alone, love does not disappear during times of hardship.

From Indigenous traditions, we learn of ancestors walking with us, of children being born with old souls, and spirits moving through wind and river and animal. In these beliefs, nothing truly dies. Everything transforms. I've seen this time and time again in the eyes of parents who have lost their child and still, somehow, continued living. They see their child in the rustle of leaves, in the butterfly that lingers, or in the dream that feels more like a visit than a memory.

Many religions and spiritual traditions understand life as a cycle—not as a straight line between birth to death, but a repeating, evolving journey. This view often brings comfort, suggesting that endings are not final, and that growth and transformation continue beyond what we can see. That the moment we are in is not the complete story.

Whether your personal expression of spirituality sits within religion or is less easily defined, the search for faith and meaning lives in the smallest of gestures. It's the kiss you place on your child's forehead, or the wish you whisper to the brightest star in the sky. It's believing you'll see your child again, even if you don't understand quite how. It's in the way you feel energy beneath your feet as you stand on the grass, and the smell of rain as it approaches. It's a belief that there is more to life than this one moment—and that parents all around the world will light candles in the dark and dare to hope.

It's acknowledging that there is one thread tying us to each other across the globe—that there are a thousand different ways to say: Even here. Even now. I will not stop loving you.

When my little one started to ask questions about death, I found myself saying something that became quite a spiritual mantra for us both. I simply said:

"My darling, I will always be your Mummy, and you will always be my baby. In this life, and the next life, and in ALL the lives that follow. We will always be together. Our love has no end."

I would like to gently acknowledge that these beliefs are not held by all—and that you may find them difficult to process, or even disagree with them on a profound level. The very nature of this conversation may bring you closer to feelings of anger than of peace. And I completely understand. If this is the case for you, please take care of yourself and move past this section. Nothing in this book is intended to offend or hurt—only to offer comfort where possible.

To the fighter,

This world we live in is so often feels like a battleground—a relentless, exhausting fight.

In the beginning, we often fight to be heard. To have the medical profession confirm what we know deep down: that something is not right with the child we know so well. Then we fight to understand what's happening, how it's happening, and what it will mean.

We fight through long nights and grief-stricken days, through emergency admissions, surgeries, and hospital stays.

We fight for better treatment options. For more time. For hope. For sleep.

Some of us fight for the life of our child. Some of us fight to keep our child alive in our hearts and minds.

We fight so hard and so long that the fight begins to live inside us. It takes up residence in our minds and our bodies. The fight becomes as big as we are. And it's exhausting.

So much of the fight is necessary—it is part of our role as our child's advocate. But some of it isn't. Some of it is simply our way of coping, of trying to wrestle back control in a world that has terrified us.

What if, instead, we surrendered some of that fight—as gracefully and calmly as we can? What if we acknowledged that so much of this is beyond our control, and we release it?

Surrendering is not giving up. It is a conscious release of the things that are weighing us down. It is done openly. Willingly. With peace.

A few years ago, I made the decision to surrender. To let go of the endless cycle of questioning every decision. That questioning had become a source of conflict—with my husband, who grew exasperated; and silently, within myself, with our medical team. It wasn't that I didn't trust them—I trust them with my life—it was that I was endlessly afraid of missing something. Something vital. Something that could change everything.

Fear was keeping me awake at night. Reading. Researching. Obsessing. And always ending up in the same place.

I was breaking my own heart.

So, one day, I made the choice to surrender. To place my trust in our incredible team, and to hand over my fear. Willingly. Calmly. Not as a defeat, but as a release.

I didn't give up. I never will.

I just chose to refocus. To reframe.

I'll still tuck my smallest worries into my pockets, and carry the bigger ones on my back—but the ones I've let go of will make the road ahead of me just a little lighter. And with a little more lightness, I can focus on what I do best: living the best life I can with my little one.

It's okay to let go.
Love, Me x

CHAPTER 12
Grief

Finding Beauty in the Broken Pieces

There is often a kind of beauty that comes with pain and suffering—a reflective knowing that life can be tough, but so are you.

The Japanese have recognised this truth and even made it into an art form over 500 years ago. Known as Kintsugi, it is a philosophy that honours resilience, transformation, and the beauty found in trauma. At its heart, Kintsugi understands that breakage and repair are part of every story—that being broken and putting ourselves back together is both ongoing and universal.

Kintsugi – the art of repairing broken pottery with gold – doesn't try to hide the cracks. It highlights them. It celebrates the journey from damaged to transformed. The once-broken piece becomes more beautiful, more valuable, because of its fractures, not despite them.

While Kintsugi has been explored by many therapists and writers, it holds particular significance for parents of critically or chronically ill children. It serves as a gentle reminder: your hardship need not be hidden. They are part of your story.

Caring for an unwell child reshapes your life in countless ways. It leaves tiny cracks in its wake. Financial stress, career setback, strained relationships, the quiet pain of siblings, fear, grief, uncertainty. These cracks can feel like shameful flaws. We often try to conceal them, believing they make us less—less stable, less worthy, less whole.

But Kintsugi teaches something else. It urges us to acknowledge the impact of our child's diagnosis—to face it with compassion, and to move forward bravely.

Imagine holding the broken pieces of your life gently in your hands, acknowledging them with grace. Imagine tending to those parts as lovingly as you care for your child. Imagine sealing each fracture with gold—a symbol of beauty, value, and strength.

Then, imagine turning back to the world—not unscarred, but whole in a new way. With golden seams that trace your emotional landscape, honouring the dance between your pain and your strength. Beauty through vulnerability. Strength in imperfection.

The Kintsugi philosophy also reminds us that vulnerability is a gateway to connection. When you acknowledge your pain, you create space for others to support you—and give them quiet permission to tend to their own broken parts, too.

Sometimes, when I sit in the paediatric oncology waiting room, I imagine gold veins tracing the surface of every person there—some bold and glimmering, others soft and fine. I see the grief that once broke us, and the courage that slowly stitched us back together. In those moments, I feel deeply proud to be among such quiet warriors.

Tip: Be brave enough to be yourself—cracks, scars, and all. In tending to your pain, remember that it is evidence of your love and your strength. You are more beautiful, more unique, for the path you've walked.

'Find me There' by Sara Rian

I am sorry for the loss of your person.
And the million things that vanished
on the day their heart stopped beating.
And the billion things you must grieve
every single day that they aren't here.
And I am sorry that there isn't a better word than just, sorry.

Losing Your Child

There are no words big enough, accurate enough, or meaningful enough to describe the grief a parent experiences when their child dies. There is simply a gaping hole in the universe, and a gaping hole in their heart.

If that heart is yours, I'm so deeply sorry for your unfathomable loss.

The thing about grief is that it is entirely personal and unique. There is no right or wrong way to experience it, and no timeframe to move through it. There is no moving past it—just moving with it, carrying it around with you as you navigate life without your child.

Therapists often reference the idea that your grief doesn't become smaller, but that over time your life grows around it, all the while accepting it as the centrepiece of your soul.

I understand that even amid future joy, there will never be a time when you're not sad that your child is gone, and it will take enormous strength to continue with your life in the rubble of your loss.

Your life without your child will forever be an intricate tapestry of emotions—a tapestry filled with pictures and colours that blind the eye with their richness. A story woven together with threads of joy, bravery, and sorrow. Love immortalised. A story the world around you needs to hear.

Keep saying their name, as will we.

Note: This book is not a guide to loss; however, there are many resources specifically designed to help you navigate the loss of your child, and you are encouraged to seek them out. Your GP, psychologist, social worker, or nurse will be able to point you in the right direction.

To the ones who are healing,

One night, as I tucked her into bed, she said to me, "Let's talk about something that makes you happier."

She'd been snuggling into me, the endlessness of her chatter a soothing balm to my heart, when she unexpectedly began to talk about the moments that had bothered her the most during 'all of this.'

She spoke calmly about being held down, arms pinned to her sides, about tubes being shoved up her nose, and the pain of it all. But not with grief, simply with acceptance. She had experienced it, named it, and shared it. Then she let it go.

I almost couldn't bear to hear it, but I smiled through too-bright eyes, holding my pain tight, like a grudge.

She talked about giving in to the general anaesthetics, not wanting to succumb and fighting it with everything she had.

"I tried not to go to sleep, but I did. Every time."

"Were you still there, Mummy, while I slept?" she asked.

And I told her, gently, that every time she closed her eyes, I would kiss her perfect cheek and whisper, "I love you, baby girl. Sleep tight."

And that as I left the room, the medical team would still be singing the words to her favourite song, their kindness bringing tears to my eyes, as they swiftly prepared the room around her sleeping body.

But that I never left, and I never will.

And she said, "that must have made you sad."

Me, sad. Not her. Me.

I imagine she saw, with her gentle soul, a little of the weight I carry, and she said, "let's talk about something that makes you happier."

My darling girl. This beautiful child who carries the universe on her shoulders and the stars in her eyes.

This sweet girl, who talks about living this life with me, and the next and the next. Who asks me to put aside her favourite dress to wear in our next life together.

Breaking my heart and mending it instantly with the force of her love. Knowing instinctively what healing looks like.

Together forever,
Me x

CHAPTER 13
Growth Through Trauma (Forged in Fire)

Growth through trauma, or post-traumatic growth (PTG), is a psychological theory that explores how individuals can experience positive changes as a result of struggling through trauma; because of what they've endured.

PTG explains how you may find a new and profound strength, wisdom, and perspective after deep hardship.

PTG is not about stepping back into who you were before the diagnosis. It's about stepping into a new, stronger, wiser version of yourself. It's not the avoidance of pain; it's transforming through it. It's an acknowledgement that it's possible to be both deeply affected by trauma and to grow from it.

A requirement of this kind of growth is that you experience the pain and the struggle, and that you find a way to make sense of the deeply challenging experience. Without the space and ability to reflect and process, healing and growth cannot occur.

You'll often hear people who have gone through a traumatic event explain that they have a greater appreciation of life, stronger emotional ties to others, and a newfound strength and resilience after moving through the healing process. This doesn't mean the deep hardship they've experienced is suddenly easy, or that they're grateful for it, but it recognises that growth and suffering can co-exist. You can be both broken and growing at the same time.

If this doesn't resonate with you yet, it's important to remember that you can be deeply affected by trauma and not grow from it—or not grow from it yet. Your ability to grow from your pain is directly linked to your ability to process it, and that ability will evolve at its own pace, at the right time for you.

The concept of PTG was first formally introduced by psychologists Richard Tedeschi and Lawrence Calhoun in the 1990s. Their research in this area was foundational, and their book "The Handbook of Posttraumatic Growth" dives deep into the science behind it.

In their research, Tedeschi and Calhoun identified five main areas where people often experience growth following trauma:

1. Appreciation for life – where you experience a deeper awareness of the preciousness of life, and a renewed gratitude for everyday moments.
2. Relationships with others – deeper, more authentic connections are formed, and you experience a greater sense of empathy for the suffering of others.
3. Personal strength – where you discover your resilience and realise that you can face whatever challenges the future throws at you.
4. New possibilities – becoming open to new opportunities and life directions as a result of re-evaluating your previous expectations.

5. Spiritual change – many people find themselves exploring spirituality, mindfulness and personal meaning, often side by side with deep questions around life and mortality.

Finding meaning and growth following trauma calls on you to embark on a journey of reflection, connection, and intentional change. To do this, you need to acknowledge not only your pain but also your growth, naming the ways in which you have developed, how your priorities have shifted, and what you may have learned about yourself. Reframing the experience is critical to growing from it.

Many people also find growth when they turn their pain into something productive or purposeful. This may look like assisting others who have faced a similar diagnosis, embarking on fundraising activities, or creating a life that feels more meaningful following diagnosis.

Tedeschi and Calhoun identify three key ways in which we find meaning:
1. The trauma shakes your core beliefs. Your child's diagnosis will very likely have disrupted your worldview, and your beliefs around safety, control and fairness may have been shattered.
2. Emotional distress and cognitive struggle - painful reflection or rumination is often a necessary part of the growth journey. Rumination is the process of deeply thinking through the situation, and can be both intrusive and unwanted, or deliberate and meaning-making.

3. Through deliberate reflection people begin to make sense of their experience and often reshape their personal story to include resilience and growth.

Deliberate reflection helps you make better sense of your experience; however, it requires you to engage in levels of emotional reflection and vulnerability that are uncomfortable to sit with.

How do you Process Trauma, Find Meaning From it, & Move Towards Growth?

Growth only occurs when you are able to process trauma, and as such, those who are willing to engage with difficult emotions by finding meaning, seeking support, and practicing self-compassion will find themselves growing and healing ahead of those who don't.

The first step in this journey is to acknowledge and accept the pain of what's happened to you, without minimising it or applying a positive filter. This stage of the healing journey isn't linear, and you must allow yourself time to grieve before you can begin to find acceptance. You can begin by being very clear about your emotions. Call them out. Name them. Instead of saying "I feel awful," say, "I feel angry because my child is so unwell, and I feel helpless to make this better." And then give yourself grace. Validate your emotions rather than downplaying them: "It makes sense that I'm feeling this way," or "This is a totally normal reaction given the situation." If you feel stuck in a pattern of negative thoughts, ask yourself whether you would talk to a close friend or loved one that way?

Rumination is the process of continuously thinking about a distressing event or painful experience in a recurring way and is an important part of processing and healing. We often hear ruminating discussed in a negative light, however positive rumination, or ruminating with intention is a critical element in your recovery. While negative rumination sees you stuck in a painful thought pattern without resolution ("why did this happen to him? Life is so cruel and unfair"), ruminating with intention, or reflecting on your pain and experience with purpose, can lead to healing. It allows personal growth through a better understanding of both the event and yourself.

Writing is a powerful way to help you process emotions and find new perspectives. Journalling or purposeful rumination can be a meaningful way to uncover emotions and buried thoughts. There are some prompts for journalling and deeper reflection in Chapter 7 (Cultivating Calm).

Exercise: write yourself a kind and compassionate letter. Begin it with: "Dear Me, I see you. You've been through so much, and I know you're hurting." Or a variation of this to suit yourself.

If you find writing difficult, dictate a voice note to yourself. Save it on your phone, and over time you'll see how much your thought patterns have changed.

Exercise: Reflect on how much has changed, from before your child's diagnosis to now. Write for 10 minutes without planning, focusing on how your perspective has shifted. This will help you identify growth and see your progress over time.

Talking is a key component to processing trauma. It allows you to integrate the experience into your life story. Trauma often gets 'stuck' in the brain's emotional centre (the amygdala), keeping you in a fight-or-flight state. When you talk about it, the prefrontal cortex (the rational thinking part of the brain) gets involved. This helps you to put words to emotions instead of just feeling overwhelmed, and gain clarity on what happened rather than reliving it chaotically. When trauma is unfolding it can often feel confused and disjointed. Talking can structure the story in a way that allows your brain to process it, and frame it in a healthier way.

Talking also helps to release emotional weight, leading to processing instead of suppressing, giving your emotions an outlet rather than trapping them in your tired body.

Telling your story is also a good way to find support and understanding from others, reminding you that you're not alone, and helping you view your experience through a kinder lens.

Exercise: Record a voice memo where you speak to yourself with the kindness and comfort that you would give a friend. Save the recording and listen to it whenever you need reassurance.

It's important to understand that the way you tell your story will shape your healing. Is your narrative fixated on the grief of the diagnosis, or on how you've changed and grown throughout the process? Notice how you tell the story and gently challenge your negative thoughts: "Her diagnosis was shocking and frightening, but I'm learning more about it every day and finding more confidence in dealing with it".

Exercise: Rewrite your story with two versions: the first where you remain stuck and helpless, and the second where you recognise your strength and growth. Which version do you want to step into?

Finding meaning in your child's diagnosis will be one of the most difficult things you will ever try to do. Finding meaning won't ease the pain, and it's critical that you acknowledge the pain will always exist, but it will help you find a place for the experience in your life story. It will allow you to reach out to others who are suffering as you have and will help you identify the things that truly matter.

Exercise: Create a meaning map. At the centre, write down your child's diagnosis. Then, around it, write down anything you've learned, strengths you've gained, new perspectives, and things you're valuing more. The thing about trauma is that it can often reveal strengths we didn't know we had.

Celebrate all growth, no matter how small it may feel, and remember that post-traumatic growth isn't about getting over your child's diagnosis, but growing with it; and despite it.

Exercise: Keep a post-traumatic stress diary. Each day, or whenever you feel like it, write down on small or large way in which you grew that day. For example:
- "I allowed myself to rest instead of continuing to research my child's condition."
- "I went for a walk and listened to my favourite podcast while someone else watched my child."

- "I laughed today as we created animals from hospital gloves."
- One of mine might be, "I heard worrying news today and didn't immediately get a migraine."

Over time, these small moments will add up to deeper transformation.

Dear me,

I know there were times you could never have imagined laughing again. That you could stand forever in the sun and never again feel its warmth. I know you stood on the ledge and stared into the abyss, wondering how you were ever going to do what needed to be done. I know you were without hope.

I know you thought you'd never step away from the ledge upon which you stood.

You couldn't imagine a future with joy, or ease, or comfort, and you didn't know how to cover your grief and be the mum you needed to be. It was hard, and it was sad, and it was terrifying. I know you woke at night in a panic, desperate and frantic, but unsure why. You carried a tightness in your chest that never let up, and there were months at a time when you couldn't get yourself together to answer the phone or keep in contact with friends. There were so many days you couldn't face the world. Because the world was too much, and pretending to be okay was too hard.

I know you were angry, and that sometimes that anger made you snap at the people you loved—because nothing was okay. You would have given everything to go back to the moment before you knew, when life was so beautiful it hurt you to look back upon it. It's okay that you were angry. You were only given 9 perfect weeks with your littlest love before finding out.

I also know the moment you decided no one could save you but yourself, and I watched you step back from the ledge and find your resolve. You turned your anger into purpose, and your fear into compassion, and started to move forward. I'm proud of you. I'm proud of you for holding your arms open for others to fall into when they received their own heartbreaking diagnoses. I'm proud of you for speaking about your experiences even though it hurt, so that our country's decision-makers can put in place better systems and structures to support those who walk alongside you, and those who are yet to come.

None of this is easy. It's still hard and sad. But there's so much joy in your world now, and so much appreciation in your heart for what you have. I see you choosing hope over fear, even when that's the more vulnerable choice. I know it wasn't an easy road to get here, but believe me when I say you're a better person for the road you've travelled.

Keep moving forward. We've got this.

With love always,
Zoë xx

CHAPTER 14
From One Parent to Another

In the midst of our own journey, we were fortunate to find support, connection, and invaluable advice from others who had walked this road before us. These words are raw, heartfelt, and real. They are gifts—from one parent to another—offered in the hope that they bring you comfort, courage, and a reminder: you are not alone.

"I love when people that have been through hell walk out of the flames carrying buckets of water for those still consumed by the fire."

—Stephanie Sparkles

Diagnosis Day: When the World Changes

"The day our whole world came crashing down. Diagnosis day. The day my life split in two. Pre diagnosis and post diagnosis."
—Amanda, mum to Ava

"Never could we imagine we would be on this side, never could we imagine we would be one of the statistics. The heartache, the pain, the fear that comes with childhood cancer is crippling."
—Aimee, mum to El

"When Ralph was diagnosed it felt as though the walls were caving in around us. I didn't know how we were going to get through this. It's what nightmares are made of and I just wanted to be able to scoop him up and be able to make it all better. It was out of my control. What I've learned from all the heartache, sadness, worry and trauma is that love prevails. The power of love, that's really what is getting us through this."
—Sophie, mum to Ralph

"No matter the diagnosis, when you look at your child, remember—they are still the same cherub they were before. What you've received is simply new information to help you better understand their world."
-Kirsty – mum to Shelby and Jackson

You are the Advocate

"Always trust your instincts. A mother knows her child best. Don't assume that your medical team will inform you of every option or give you the full picture when it comes to major decisions affecting your child's future. Take the time to do your own research and advocate for your child with everything you've got. If you don't speak up for them, who will?"
—Sammie, mum to Luna

"Question everything. Mums know their kids best. If you don't feel like you're being heard, speak up and don't be afraid to ask for second opinions."
—Lauren

"Don't stress and overthink, it won't help. Until you get the plan. When you get the plan, work the plan. When the plan stops working, go back and get a new plan."
—SJ Thompson, mum to OS warrior Rayne

"Be your child's advocate no matter what! The medical team knows medically what to do. You know what your child needs you to do. Together more positive things will happen!"
- Bianca, mum to Addison

"Strive for Thrivorship, from the day of diagnosis. At the moment, in Australia, the goal is for the child simply to survive.

One in five children are still stolen by the beast, and some diagnoses have a zero percent five-year event free survival (EFS) which is totally unacceptable. Our children deserve the opportunity to thrive with cancer, through treatment and beyond. They desperately need access to (and funding for) all the evidence based allied health offerings to support their minds, bodies and spirits. And for families too, who are both the frontline and backbone of their child's treatment protocol, forevermore."

- Nic Kennedy, oncology mumma and fierce advocate

"The best advice any of us can give is - become the biggest and loudest advocate for your child, because if you don't, who will? Trust your gut, if something doesn't feel right, ask questions and keep asking until you get answers."

- SJ Thompson, mum to OS warrior Rayne

"I'd like for parents to know to advocate for your child fiercely. Don't be afraid to speak up.
And respect your nurses - they are angels."

- Raffa's mum and dad

Moments That Stay With You

"Lean on your nurses for support and advice. I'll never forget our nurse, when Ethan had sepsis and the doctors were still figuring out what to do, saying, 'I'm not losing him on my watch,' as she wheeled in the crash cart."

—Janine, mum to Ethan

"When Luna was first diagnosed with stage 4 high-risk neuroblastoma, she wasn't even two years old at the time. We were thrust immediately into treatment. The shock of the diagnosis barely had time to settle before we were already in the trenches. One thing I wish her medical team had told us is that it was possible to preserve her eggs, so that if she wanted to have biological children later in life, she could. Unfortunately, no one informed us about this option... Cancer already takes so much from our children, and this is just another piece of Luna's future that it has stolen."

—Sammie, mum to Luna

Grief Within the Journey

"One of the hardest things I felt when Laylah was first diagnosed is that I was grieving the loss of a child, even though she was still with us. I didn't know how to cope with that feeling. I didn't know if I was the only one who felt like that... or how to overcome it."

—Emma, mum to Laylah

"Sometimes I feel like I have this contagious disease called never-ending grief that makes people uncomfortable and awkward with me too, not knowing what to say or just not saying anything at all."

—Amanda, mum to Ava

"There are some griefs you never really get over. You absorb them and on your best days they make you mighty. On other days they threaten to fell you to your knees. There are still days that I fall to my knees. I think there always will be and that feels a lot like recovery too. Recovery to me is crying often and openly. It's saying no to what I know will burden me at times I can't carry it."

—Tanya, mum to Lara

"As a mum, it's devastating to watch my child battle a disease that's not well-known, resulting in feelings of isolation and limited upport. It makes everyday conversations and navigating systems like the health system, and even sporting code classification systems, incredibly challenging. While Grayson may look normal to society now, what lies beneath is the darkness that shadows his future."

—Jen, mum to Grayson

Support & Connection

"When Addison was first diagnosed, it was a bit of a whirlwind for us. They didn't quite know what exactly she had and then there were also a lot of tests to confirm the reason for her severe plastic anaemia. I found, at first, that everyone was very attentive friends wise. A lot of people wanting to do a lot of things for you - meal trains there to send you things and assist you. But as the treatments went on, everyone gets back to their own lives. You are all still battling the same battles at the beginning just not with as much attention and help from others. And like I said everyone has their own lives they've got their own problems. It was just, for me, we had a lot of people at the beginning when we didn't even know what was going on. I think really it started to feel lonelier the further we went into treatment."

—Bianca, mum to Addison

"You'll form some of your closest friendships in the most unexpected places. For example, my friend Christa has been a blessing, the biggest cheerleader and the best friend during our journey, all while navigating her own son's journey. We met in the laundry room of all places!"

—Sammie, mum to Luna

"Before you think of ghosting someone under the guise of not wanting to bother them or not knowing what to say—remember we don't care what you say. We want to know we aren't alone. We also have to continue on with life. It's nice to feel like some parts of our world haven't changed."

—Aimee, mum to Elkie

"When Mitchell was first diagnosed, I felt utterly crushed. Whenever someone asked how I was coping, my default response was always, "It is what it is," or simply, "I'm fine." In truth, I wasn't fine at all. When I tried to express my deepest fears and concerns, I was often met with well-meaning but dismissive reassurances—phrases like, "He's a fighter," "He's got this," "He looks so good," or "You'd never even know he had cancer." While I understood the intent behind those words, they often made me want to scream. In those moments, I didn't need positivity I needed space to be honest about the fear, the uncertainty, and the pain we were living through."

—Alyce, mum to Mitchell

"I wanted to retreat, to shut myself off from the world. It felt like the only way to protect myself, to handle the weight of it all."

—Hayley Smith, mum to Elsey-Rae,
and co-founder of Cancer Dancer

Coping & Self-Care

"When you're taking care of a loved one on their cancer journey, the words 'make time for self-care' can feel frustrating. Between appointments, caregiving tasks, and the emotional rollercoaster that defines each day, it feels impossible to carve out a moment for yourself."
—Hayley Smith, mum to Elsey-Rae,
and co-founder of Cancer Dancer

"Find solitude in the shower and cry it all out."
—Janine, mum to Ethan

"Whether it is a yoga class, a walk, a hike or just some gentle stretching—moving with intention changes your frequency. The energy transforms how you are showing up for yourself and what you radiate out."
—Hayley Smith, mum to Elsey-Rae,
and co-founder of Cancer Dancer

"Get psychological help in the beginning, before you start to lose yourself and your mental health gets bad as a parent. I sent myself to a dark place constantly looking up chances of relapses which is completely out of anyone's control."
—Kelly, mum to Mileah

"Recovery is feeling safe to be fragile, it's sharing with friends and colleagues when I'm on shaky ground. Recovery is trusting happiness, trusting hope, and it's wholeheartedly trusting my friendships and myself."

—Tanya, mum to Lara

"It's ok to not be everything to everyone, even to your sick child. It takes a village. You can't meet everyone's expectations of what you should do and how you should handle it/ behaviour. No one knows what it is like. Even parents in a similar situation it's still different. I don't regret how we handle the situation. I just wish I would have been kinder to myself."

—Samantha – mum to Annabelle

Healing, Growth & Hope

"Opening up to life again has been an extraordinary journey of growth for us all. It was a path we never could have walked without experiencing loss. Learning to feel alive again, despite the grief, has been a powerful process."

—Hayley Smith, mum to Elsey-Rae,

and co-founder of Cancer Dancer

"Along your journey, you may hear labels connected to diagnoses. It can be painful to hear them, but remember, you are important in this journey, and whatever you are feeling is valid."

—Kirsty, mum to Shelby and Jackson

"Make friends! Oncology ward is full of different stories, but similar struggles! Also, remember, it's a rollercoaster!!! It's emotional!!! When everyone else is starting to heal, remember you will also need to. Remember you are so amazing!!! Your child will know that the most!!!"

—Bianca, mum to Addison

"Zoe, I remember when we were sitting together. We were both nursing coffee and I was nursing a new PTSD diagnosis. I said, 'I don't want to feel like this. I'm turning this into Post Traumatic Growth'. You said to me 'How will you know when that happens?' and I answered, 'When I no longer feel like this.' Recovery looks nothing like I would have liked it to. It's more fragile than I'd hoped. Recovery looks a lot like starting again after setbacks, without shame or blame. Recovery feels honest, and clean, and it brings with it a feeling of connection to others I would have been terrified of when my poor, battered heart was broken."

—Tanya, mum to Lara

Practical Advice

"When you're in hospital, put a blanket down under the sheet when making your bed. Those hospital mattresses get really cold about 2am and if you don't, you'll wake up with the sorest back."

—SJ Thompson, mum to OS warrior Rayne

"Don't stress about missing school! I've spent so much time and energy stressing about this. Due to anxiety, we made the decision to homeschool this year. I've quickly realised how little work is actually done during a school day (we cover the same in less than 2 hrs). After reflecting on everything Seth did learn while going through treatment and having discussions with his teacher from last year it's evident that the 8ish months he was away from school did not negatively impact his education."

—Beck, mum to Seth

"My top tip: A head torch for reading in bed once your child has gone to sleep but you're wide awake and you don't want to wake them up! Also, make up a list of things you would appreciate friends and family doing when they don't know how to help - making frozen meals, doing laundry, taking pets for a walk, mowing the lawn. These could also be gifts to give, for example to pay for a cleaner/gardening service etc."

—Tracey, mum to Evie

"Bills and cost of things rack up! Get a GoFundMe! No you're not begging! Sadly you're not being looked after enough, and luckily real people out there will help!"

—Bianca, mum to Addison

"We always had a hospital bag packed and ready to go during Emme's chemo. Inside, we kept the essentials: warm socks, phone and iPad chargers, tea and coffee bags, a reusable coffee cup with a lid, pain relief (for those sneaky hospital headaches), and a long-lasting snack like a protein or muesli bar, as well as some colouring-in activities for Emme —especially helpful during long Emergency admissions. We also included basic toiletries, hand cream, lip balm, tissues and at least one vomit bag. When fevers spiked and I knew an admission was inevitable, I'd pack a second bag with my kindle, some warm, comfy clothes (hospital rooms are always so cold!) and a few last-minute things—like whatever food Emme was currently tolerating. Our ever-ready hospital bag came from hard-won experience, and it meant we never had to worry about forgetting the essentials in the rush to get to the hospital."

—Zoe, mum to Emme

Thank you to every parent who shared their story, their grief, and their grit. Your words are a lifeline to those still in the fire.

Author's Note

If you've made it to this page, I want to say thank you. Thank you for walking with me through the mess and the meaning, the heartbreak and the hope. Writing Life Interrupted was never about having the answers—it was about creating a companion for the journey. A place where you could come and feel less alone.

I know this isn't the story any of us would have chosen. No one wants to hold their child's hand through pain, uncertainty, or a diagnosis that changes everything. But here we are—still breathing, still showing up, still loving with all we have. That, in itself, is extraordinary.

This book began as scribbled notes and quiet conversations with other parents who understood what words often can't express. It became a collection of hard-earned lessons and small, sacred truths. I hope it has offered you some comfort, a little clarity, or simply the sense that someone else gets it.

If there's one thing I hope you take from these pages, it's this: you are doing better than you think. You are strong, even on the days you feel like you're falling apart. And your love—fierce, flawed, unwavering—is enough.

I don't know how your story will unfold from here. But I do know that you are not alone. There is a quiet army of parents walking this path beside you—tired, tender, and brave in ways they never asked to be. I'm one of them.

From one interrupted life to another—thank you for letting me be part of your journey.

With love, Zoë x

Appendix

Questions you may ask yourself or others may ask of you:

1. **What does this diagnosis mean?** Ask for a simple, easy to understand explanation of what the condition is.
2. **Is the condition life-threatening, life-limiting or life-changing?** This is a painful question but can help contextualise the current moment and the future.
3. **What causes this condition?** Understanding the underlying causes can be useful in understanding what's happening. It may also provide you with relevant information regarding your other children, particularly if the condition is genetic.
4. **Is it common?** Knowing this information can help steer you towards support groups and connect with others in the same boat.
5. **Could our other children have the same condition?** Is it genetic? If so, how do we test our other children?
6. **Is the condition curable, or will it need ongoing management?** This helps set realistic expectations about the intensity of care.
7. **What are the short and long-term implications of the diagnosis?** What are the symptoms, complications, etc.

8. **Does my child need treatment?** What would that look like? Are there options? Would treatment be ongoing or for a period of time?
9. **What are the risks of treatment, or the risks of not treating?** And is it a choice, or essential? Do you have time to think it through?
10. **What are the short and long-term side effects of treatment?**
11. **How will this impact my child's life, at home, at school, during play, and sport?** Will they be able to continue these things, or will they need to stop? Will they need time in hospital?
12. **What are the warning signs we should watch out for that might indicate our child's condition is worsening?** Understanding when to bring your child in for medical assessment is imperative. Knowing when to worry and when not to worry will become a big part of your journey.
13. **How should we talk to our child about their diagnosis?**
14. **How do we talk to their siblings?** Your medical practitioner should be able to refer you to a social worker or counsellor to help ensure you're supported when talking to your child and siblings. If they don't, ask the following question:
15. **Is there someone who can support us through this?** This might be a charity organisation, a social worker, or a nurse, for example.
16. **Are there any educational resources you can recommend?** Learning from the most up-to-date medical information that's specific to your child's condition is invaluable.
17. **Are there specialist services we will need to see?** Will there be a team of specialists? How often will we see them? How do I organise this?

18. **Will you be managing our child's ongoing care?** You may be receiving this news from a specialist who will continue to manage your child's health, or from your GP who might refer you to the relevant specialist(s).
19. **What costs should we expect, and what is covered by insurance or by the government?** Knowing the expected financial impact will better prepare you for the future.
20. **What are our next immediate steps?** What happens now?
21. **Who can we contact if we have any concerns or further questions?**
22. **How will this diagnosis affect our daily life as a family?** This can help parents anticipate changes to routines, work, childcare, or other responsibilities.
23. **How can we support our child emotionally and mentally through this?** Understanding what psychological support may be needed can help foster resilience and well-being for the child
24. **Are there parent/carer support groups you recommend?** Connecting with others who are going through something similar can be incredibly grounding and affirming.
25. **What should we record or track at home?** Keeping track of symptoms, medications, or side effects can help with ongoing care and communication with doctors.
26. **Is there someone who can help us coordinate care and appointments?** Some hospitals or clinics offer care coordinators or case managers, which can reduce overwhelm.
27. **What should we do in an emergency?** Having a clear plan for emergencies (e.g., who to call, where to go) gives parents confidence and a sense of control.

28. **Will my child need special equipment or accommodations at home, school, or elsewhere?** It's helpful to address this early in the diagnosis, even if the answer is "not right now."

Acknowledgement

So many people have contributed to our medical and emotional journey over the past ten years, and in doing so, have helped shape the words within this book. While it's impossible to acknowledge everyone who has played a part, please know that I carry your impact with deep gratitude.

Firstly, to the extraordinary parents who shared their stories and insights with unflinching honesty - thank you. Your words are woven through these pages, and your courage has shaped the heart of this work. I am humbled by your generosity and honoured to carry pieces of your journeys here. A big thank you also to the Qld Paediatric Oncology Support Village – the most beautiful group that none of us ever expected to be a part of.

To the dedicated caregivers, nurses, doctors, and staff at the Queensland Children's Hospital—especially those who have looked after our daughter with such compassion and skill—thank you for the countless ways you bring comfort, dignity, and care to children and their families. Your presence in our lives has made more of a difference than words can express.

In particular, thank you to Dr Tony Prado, who sat before me in 2015 and delivered the unthinkable confirmation that Emme has NF1. I can't imagine how hard it was for you to do that, and I'm so grateful that you delivered the news with such kindness and humanity. All these years later, I haven't forgotten a single moment of that day. Also, to Dr Adriane Sinclair and Dr John Down: thank you for going the extra mile to make things easier for Emme. Your kindness means the world to us. Thank you to Dr Sonia Yuen, who held Emme as a tiny baby in such capable hands, and who has gently reminded me over the years to treasure the moments and to prioritise my emotional wellbeing.

An extra-special thank you to Dr Tim Hassall, our daughter's oncologist—thank you for your extraordinary care, your calm presence, and the depth of your commitment. Your work changes lives every single day, and ours is one of them. Thank you for the bond you've created with Emme, and for enabling her to live a full and happy life.

To our Clinical Nurse Coordinator, Brooke—who's walked alongside us from the early days of explaining central lines and chemo with a giant Elmo doll (I'm sorry I cried so much I had to steal the tissue box from reception) to the conversations of now, which are so rich and varied—from treatment, to life, travel, and family. Your honesty, compassion, and kindness will never be forgotten.

We're indebted to our Allied Health team (Shannon, Kristy, Emily, Julian and Anna), past and present, who support us daily to ensure Emme is happy, strong and capable. Thank you for your passion and commitment. Heartfelt thanks to Shannon—for your insight and experience that helped shape parts of this book, and for everything you are to both Emme and me.

To the Children's Tumour Foundation of Australia (past and present - Ruth, Meredith, Leanne, Renee, Nat, Louise, Richard and so many more) – thank you. Your care, friendship and support has been invaluable. The work you do is meaningful to so many. Extra special thanks to John Hughes, whose personal commitment to ending NF means everything. To Redkite, who provided us with emotional support when we needed it most, and to Make-A-Wish, for the beautiful memories.

To our family—I know this journey has broken you at times too. It's not been an easy road, and certainly not one any of us could have expected. Thank you for your love and support towards Emme when she's needed it most. And to my mum, who has heard almost every painful thought I've ever had and carried it with such grace and love. Sorry about that! I deeply appreciate your unwavering presence and strength. I know how hard it's been, and I couldn't do it without you.

To my friends... I would be lost without you. You inspired me to write about unicorns and to shine a light on the immense love that exists in the world, even amidst grief. Especially in grief. Jo and Juanita, thank you always—for being literal and figurative unicorns in our lives. For tiny nails painted on hospital beds, and the boys ferried to school so I could be with Emme. To Sara and Nerissa, for the memes, the jokes, the constant check-ins, and the love. We became friends when you left food on my doorstep. To Lauren F, for your friendship in those terrifying early days, and to Rachel and Bec for sharing the early days of diagnosis (for us all) with tears and laughter. And to the Bedroom Makeover Crew and everyone who contributed to make the kids so happy. To my school BFFs—your food deliveries and care parcels brought me to tears. And to Storrm and Kirsty—we'll always have Hawaii.

To Tanya, for vegemite, tears and a soul connection. I hate that you know this world so well, but love that it led me to you. To Eliza, for your endless generosity—whether it was donuts, meals, gifts for Emme, or the offer of a weekend away—you are amazing. To Nath, who sat with me mid-renovation, mid-chemo, and tried to get me to eat cupcakes. To Crackerjack Jo, for your friendship and for endlessly spoiling Emme. To our Noosa crew—Jo, James, Juanita, Matt, Kerri and Dave—for giving us something to look forward to each year, and for the human pyramids on the beach. To Cristi, who never gave up on me, even when I stopped answering the phone. To Justine, who organised for Emme to meet the love of her life, Hugh Jackman. To Kristy, for wanting to understand how to help her friends who were hurting. And to Janine—I wish I could change all of this for you, and that our friendship didn't span both the real world and the oncology world.

To Crystal Leonardi from Bowerbird Publishing—thank you for your insight and guidance in shaping this manuscript into its truest form. Your clarity and care have been invaluable. It was a pleasure to work with you.

And lastly, the hardest acknowledgment of all. Nic, Harry, and Emme—no words can fully capture what you mean to me. So instead, I'll continue to show you daily how grateful I am, how proud I am, and how much I love you. And to my husband, what a journey it's been. Only you and I truly know what we've endured. I love you.

To all those who have walked in and out of our lives over the past decade—thank you. There are so many people I haven't mentioned by name who matter deeply.

This book is for all who have ever felt the world tilt beneath them and still found the grace to keep going.

With deep gratitude,
Zoë

From the Publisher

In Life Interrupted, author Zoë Rehbein offers an extraordinary blend of honest, practical guidance, and unwavering compassion for parents navigating the unthinkable: the diagnosis of a serious medical condition in their child. Drawing deeply from her own lived experience and years of advocacy, Zoë has crafted a resource that feels like a lifeline—steady, empathetic, and real.

There is no sugar-coating here, but neither is their despair. Instead, Zoë meets parents in the eye of the storm with grace and understanding, acknowledging the tidal wave of emotions—shock, fear, anger, grief—that follow a diagnosis, while offering clear, compassionate steps to survive and eventually, to find meaning in the chaos.

Zoë's writing is beautifully clear, emotionally intelligent, and often poetic in its simplicity. Readers will come away not only with tools for survival but with a deeper understanding of the strength that can emerge through suffering. This is a book that validates pain while gently encouraging transformation—a rare and precious combination.

Congratulations Zoë, Life Interrupted was a gift to publish. I wish you all the best in your new journey as a published author and hope Life Interrupted is the tool that will help countless families.

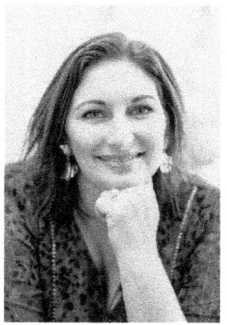

Crystal Leonardi
Bowerbird Publishing
www.crystalleonardi.com

www.ingramcontent.com/pod-product-compliance
Lightning Source LLC
Chambersburg PA
CBHW042319090526
44583CB00025BA/3158